Specialty Competencies in
Clinical Neuropsychology

Series in Specialty Competencies in Professional Psychology

TITLES IN THE SERIES

Specialty Competencies in School Psychology, Rosemary Flanagan *and* Jeffrey A. Miller

Specialty Competencies in Organizational and Business Consulting Psychology, Jay C. Thomas

Specialty Competencies in Geropsychology, Victor Molinari (Ed.)

Specialty Competencies in Forensic Psychology, Ira K. Packer *and* Thomas Grisso

Specialty Competencies in Couple and Family Psychology, Mark Stanton *and* Robert Welsh

Specialty Competencies in Clinical Child and Adolescent Psychology, Alfred J. Finch, Jr., John E. Lochman, W. Michael Nelson III, *and* Michael C. Roberts

Specialty Competencies in Clinical Neuropsychology, Greg J. Lamberty *and* Nathaniel W. Nelson

GREG J. LAMBERTY
NATHANIEL W. NELSON

Specialty Competencies in
Clinical Neuropsychology

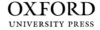

OXFORD
UNIVERSITY PRESS

OXFORD
UNIVERSITY PRESS

Oxford University Press, Inc., publishes works that further
Oxford University's objective of excellence
in research, scholarship, and education.

Oxford   New York
Auckland   Cape Town   Dar es Salaam   Hong Kong   Karachi
Kuala Lumpur   Madrid   Melbourne   Mexico City   Nairobi
New Delhi   Shanghai   Taipei   Toronto

With offices in
Argentina   Austria   Brazil   Chile   Czech Republic   France   Greece
Guatemala   Hungary   Italy   Japan   Poland   Portugal   Singapore
South Korea   Switzerland   Thailand   Turkey   Ukraine   Vietnam

Copyright © 2012 by Oxford University Press, Inc.

Published by Oxford University Press, Inc.
198 Madison Avenue, New York, New York 10016
www.oup.com

Oxford is a registered trademark of Oxford University Press

Library of Congress Cataloging-in-Publication Data

Lamberty, Gregory J.
Specialty competencies in clinical neuropsychology / Greg J. Lamberty, Nathaniel W. Nelson.
p. ; cm. — (Series in specialty competencies in professional psychology)
Includes bibliographical references and index.
ISBN 978-0-19-538744-5
1. Clinical neuropsychology. 2. Clinical competence. I. Nelson, Nathaniel W. II. Title.
III. Series: Series in specialty competencies in professional psychology.
[DNLM: 1. Clinical Medicine—methods. 2. Neuropsychology. 3. Clinical Competence. WL 103.5]
RC386.6.N48L36 2012
616.8—dc23
                                                                                        2011026863

Printed in the United States of America
on acid-free paper

To Laurie, my amazing partner and best friend.
You are my inspiration.
GJL

For my wife, Rebecca,
the joy and love of my life.
NWN

ABOUT THE SERIES IN SPECIALTY COMPETENCIES IN PROFESSIONAL PSYCHOLOGY

This series is intended to describe state-of-the-art functional and foundational competencies in professional psychology across extant and emerging specialty areas. Each book in this series provides a guide to best practices across both core and specialty competencies as defined by a given professional psychology specialty.

The impetus for this series was created by various growing movements in professional psychology during the past 15 years. First, as an applied discipline, psychology is increasingly recognizing the unique and distinct nature among a variety of orientations, modalities, and approaches with regard to professional practice. These specialty areas represent distinct ways of practicing one's profession across various domains of activities that are based on distinct bodies of literature and often addressing differing populations or problems. For example, the American Psychological Association (APA) in 1995 established the Commission on the Recognition of Specialties and Proficiencies in Professional Psychology (CRSPPP) in order to define criteria by which a given specialty could be recognized. The Council of Credentialing Organizations in Professional Psychology (CCOPP), an inter-organizational entity, was formed in reaction to the need to establish criteria and principles regarding the types of training pro-grams related to the education, training, and professional development of individuals seeking such specialization. In addition, the Council on Specialties in Professional Psychology (COS) was formed in 1997, indepen-dent of APA, to foster communication among the established specialties, in order to offer a unified position to the pubic regarding specialty education and training, credentialing, and practice standards across specialty areas.

Simultaneously, efforts to actually define professional competence regarding psychological practice have also been growing significantly. For example, the APA-sponsored Task Force on Assessment of Competence in Professional Psychology put forth a series of guiding principles for the assessment of competence within professional psychology, based, in part, on a review of competency assessment models developed both within (e.g., Assessment of Competence Workgroup from Competencies Conference—Roberts et al., 2005) and outside (e.g., Accreditation Council for Graduate Medical Education and American Board of Medical Specialties, 2000) the profession of psychology (Kaslow et al., 2007).

Moreover, additional professional organizations in psychology have provided valuable input into this discussion, including various associations primarily interested in the credentialing of professional psychologists, such as the American Board of Professional Psychology (ABPP), the Association of State and Provincial Psychology Boards (ASPBB), and the National Register of Health Service Providers in Psychology. This widespread interest and importance of the issue of competency in professional psychology can be especially appreciated given the attention and collaboration afforded to this effort by international groups, including the Canadian Psychological Association and the International Congress on Licensure, Certification, and Credentialing in Professional Psychology.

Each volume in the series is devoted to a specific specialty and provides a definition, description, and development timeline of that specialty, including its essential and characteristic pattern of activities, as well as its distinctive and unique features. Each set of authors, long-term experts, and veterans of a given specialty, were asked to describe that specialty along the lines of both functional and foundational competencies. *Functional competencies* are those common practice activities provided at the specialty level of practice that include, for example, the application of its science base, assessment, intervention, consultation, and where relevant, supervision, management, and teaching. *Foundational competencies* represent core knowledge areas which are integrated and cut across all functional competencies to varying degrees, and dependent upon the specialty, in various ways. These include ethical and legal issues, individual and cultural diversity considerations, interpersonal interactions, and professional identification.

Whereas we realize that each specialty is likely to undergo changes in the future, we wanted to establish a baseline of basic knowledge and principles that comprise a specialty highlighting both its commonalities with other areas of professional psychology, as well as its distinctiveness. We look forward to seeing the dynamics of such changes, as well as the emergence of new specialties in the future.

In this volume, Lamberty and Nelson have taken on the difficult challenge of succinctly describing the foundational and functional competencies related to the broad field of clinical neuropsychology. Whereas the beginning roots of this specialty can be found in fields over six to seven decades old, it has grown very rapidly during the past 20–30 years.

Increasingly, more and more doctoral programs in clinical psychology, as well as predoctoral internship programs, have developed concentrations in this area, as the need for predoctoral training in this specialty becomes increasingly acknowledged. Typically thought of as the professional application of areas related to brain-behavior relationships, it is firmly grounded in psychology, behavioral neurology, psychiatry, psychometrics, and statistics. These authors do a superb job in distilling not only the most important dimensions of the current science and practice related to clinical neuropsychology, but also delineate important future directions and challenges. Those readers interested in obtaining a firm grasp of past influences, the extant literature, knowledge about important professional issues, and an appreciation of the myriad future possibilities related to this specialty will be delighted to find them all here in this single volume.

Arthur M. Nezu
Christine Maguth Nezu

References

Kaslow et al. (2007). Guiding principles and recommendations for the assessment of competence. *Professional Psychology: Research and Practice, 38*, 441–451.

Roberts et al. (2005). Fostering a culture shift: Assessment of competence in the education and careers of professional psychologists. *Professional Psychology: Research and Practice, 36*, 355–361.

CLINICAL NEUROPSYCHOLOGY TIMELINE

1879   W. Wundt establishes the first laboratory of psychology at the University of Leipzig

1885   F. Galton establishes the *Anthropometric Laboratory* in London

1905   The *Binet Simon Scale* is published as first usable intelligence measure

1916   L. Terman develops the *Stanford Binet* (English revision of the Binet Simon Scale)

1917   Army *Alpha* and *Beta* tests are developed

1939   D. Wechsler publishes the *Wechsler-Bellevue* intelligence test

1947   W. Halstead publishes *Biological Intelligence*

1955   R. Reitan adapts and extends Halstead's measures to develop the *Halstead Reitan Neuropsychological Test Battery*

1967   International Neuropsychological Society established

1975   A.-L. Christensen publishes *Luria's neuropsychological investigation.*

1979   H. Goodglass & E. Kaplan describe the methods of what will later become known as the *Boston Process Approach* to neuropsychological assessment

1980   APA's Division 40 – Clinical Neuropsychology established

1987   INS/Division 40 Task Force on Education, Accreditation and Credentialing offers guidelines for training programs

1989   Division 40 approves Definition of a Clinical Neuropsychologist

1996   APA's Committee for the Recognition of Specialties and Proficiencies in Professional Psychology recognizes Clinical Neuropsychology as a specialty

1997   Houston Conference on specialty education and training in Clinical Neuropsychology convenes and produces a model of specialty training in clinical neuropsychology

2001   National Academy of Neuropsychology approves Definition of a Clinical Neuropsychologist

2007   American Academy of Clinical Neuropsychology publishes Practice Guidelines for Neuropsychological Assessment and Consultation

2011   The Clinical Neuropsychology Synarchy works toward more comprehensive guidelines for clinical neuropsychology practice

CONTENTS

PART I   Introduction to Clinical Neuropsychology Practice in Professional Psychology

ONE   Conceptual and Scientific Foundations of Clinical Neuropsychology   3

TWO   Professional Practice of Clinical Neuropsychology   13

PART II   Functional Competency — Assessment

THREE   Assessment Strategies   33

FOUR   Case Formulation in Clinical Neuropsychology   44

PART III   Functional Competency — Report Writing

FIVE   The Neuropsychological Evaluation Report   63

PART IV   Other Functional Competencies — Intervention

SIX   Intervention and Consultation in Clinical Neuropsychology   85

PART V   Foundational Competencies

SEVEN   Ethical Standards of Practice in Neuropsychology   99

EIGHT   Future Directions   114

Appendices

A. Reports of the INS/Division 40 Task Force on Education, Accreditation, and Credentialing   125

B. Division 40 (1989): Definition of a Clinical Neuropsychologist   131

C. Public Description of Clinical Neuropsychology from the APA Council for the Recognition of Specialties and Proficiencies in Professional Psychology (CRSPPP)   132

D. *The Houston Conference on Specialty Education
and Training in Clinical Neuropsychology
Policy Statement*   134

E. *National Academy of Neuropsychology Approved
Definition of a Clinical Neuropsychologist*   142

F. *American Academy of Clinical Neuropsychology
(AACN) Practice Guidelines for Neuropsychological
Assessment and Consultation*   144

References   168

Key Terms   183

Index   185

About the Authors   193

About the Series Editors   195

PART I

Introduction to Clinical Neuropsychology Practice in Professional Psychology

ONE

Conceptual and Scientific Foundations of Clinical Neuropsychology

Clinical neuropsychology is a specialty practice area that has evolved gradually over the past 50 to 60 years, but even more rapidly in the past two to three decades (Boake, 2008). It is typically asserted that neuropsychology is the study of brain-behavior relationships. While the phrasing of that popular definition sounds succinct, the subject matter is almost indescribably broad. Such a definition is also insufficient for those interested in a description of a clinical specialty. In the course of a specialty's development, many changes occur and result in an eventual need for clear standardization of education, training, experience, and credentialing processes. In concert with practitioner definitions, guidelines and standards regarding the practice field itself must also emerge. These processes have been particularly active in clinical neuropsychology in the past 10 to 20 years (APA CRSPPP, 2010; Heilbronner, 2007; INS/Division 40, 1987; NAN, 2001).

As a specialty field, neuropsychology is rather young, but its roots are deep. Organizations tend to develop when a field achieves a critical mass of people who share an identity based on their interests, duties, and sense of purpose. This has been true of clinical neuropsychology at least since the mid-1960s in the United States.

A review of some historical background is in order before current definitions of the specialty of clinical neuropsychology are presented (see chapter 2). Clinical neuropsychology is a hybrid enterprise that requires background and knowledge in the clinical fields of neurology and psychiatry, clinical psychology, psychometrics, and cognitive psychology. The modern histories of these fields date back more than two hundred years. Sources of information about the history of neuroscience abound, especially given the ease of internet searching. Stanley Finger (2001; 2005) has been among the most ambitious historians in this area, and his Oxford University Press books are an excellent resource for biographical sketches and summaries of important issues of the day.

Clinical Medicine Influences

Thomas Willis (1621–1675) is often referred to as the founder of neurology for his work dating back to the seventeenth century. He coined the term *neurology* in the course of his exhaustive work on the anatomy of the brain and subsequent examinations of the clinical correlates of pathology of the nervous system (Zimmer, 2004). Prior to that time, understanding of the role of the brain in human cognition was limited by observation and theorizing based on the medico-religious traditions of the Middle Ages. Dissection and other anatomical methods were not widely practiced by scientists and physicians, particularly with human subjects, thus leaving discovery of such relationships to those who dared to—quite literally— look deeper into their subject matter.

John Hughlings Jackson (1835–1911) is widely regarded as one of the most important clinical thinkers in the history of neurology. He championed the now well understood idea that mental functions are localizable to different parts of the brain. Jackson's observations of his wife's epilepsy led him to suggest that seizures were caused by electrical discharges that began in a specific part of the brain and moved throughout the brain in a manner that could be understood by careful description of the behavioral aspects of a seizure (Finger, 2001). His theories predated animal cortical stimulation studies by Eduard Hitzig (1838–1907) and Gustav Fritsch (1837–1927), and subsequent work by his colleague David Ferrier (1843–1928). This work helped to establish the fact that there were clear structure-to-function relationships in mammalian brains (Finger, 2005).

In this same time frame, important clinico-anatomical work by Paul Broca (1824–1880), Karl Wernicke (1848–1905), and others laid the foundation for localization theories in humans, and have stood the test of time. Broca and Wernicke conducted important postmortem investigations in patients with well-characterized clinical features and showed conclusively that pathology in specific brain regions was clearly associated with distinct patterns of clinical dysfunction (Finger, 2001; 2005).

Arguably the most famous and influential figures in fin de siècle neurology and psychiatry were Jean-Martin Charcot (1825–1893) and Sigmund Freud (1856–1939). As a student of Charcot's, Freud began to develop his theory of psychoanalysis when working with hysteria patients at the Salpetriere in Paris. The theoretical directions taken by Freud and Charcot diverged, but an understanding that the cause of mental or psychiatric illness was fundamentally biological was shared.

The import of these early clinical theories for the field of neuropsychology is clear. The brain is the organ of behavior, and damage to or derangements in brain function are likely to result in abnormalities or deficits in behavior, broadly construed (Finger, 2001; 2005). The corpus of cases undergirding neurology grew substantially in the nineteenth and early twentieth centuries and included eponymous contributions by luminaries such as Babinski, Broca, Charcot, Friedreich, L'hermitte, Oppenheim, Romberg, and Wernicke. Careful case descriptions provided the foundation for future generations' understanding of increasingly sublime "diseases" of the mind. However, these early clinical pioneers lacked systematized and data-driven methods for quantifying these observations. The earliest experimental and physiological psychologists stepped into the breach to add data and rigorous methodology to the picture, and the empirical examination of the mind began in earnest (Finger, 2001).

Psychometric Influences

During the nineteenth century several figures were involved in quantifying specific abilities, leading to the study of individual differences or *psychometrics*. Among the earliest and most notable of these characters was Francis Galton (1822–1911), whose numerous contributions to mathematics, statistics, and psychometrics formed the basis for experimentation with and assessment of human abilities. Galton was a brilliant experimenter and devised many different measures for quantifying human abilities. In true empirical fashion, he collected data on a host of tasks that, to the casual observer, may have said little about the essence of human strengths or limitations (Bulmer, 2003). His anthropometric laboratory collected data on tasks that are similar to the early staples of neuropsychological assessment. In addition to measuring all manner of body characteristics, Galton was particularly interested in sensory abilities (vision, audition, tactile senses, and appreciation of differences) and how they differed among individuals (Galton, 1879—a focus that would be evident in the work of Europe's early experimental psychologists.

Galton frequently pointed out the importance of objective measurement. His work presages modern scientific and neuropsychological thinking. A comment from an early article in the journal *Brain* is reminiscent of today's prevailing attitudes about the nature of scientific knowledge and expertise. Galton stated that "until the phenomena of any branch of knowledge have been subjected to measurement and number, it cannot assume the status and dignity of a science" (Galton, 1879). Such measurement is the stuff of modern neuropsychological practice.

Karl Pearson (1857–1936) was a mathematician who studied with Galton at the University College London in the late 1800s and early 1900s. He was instrumental in developing the statistical concepts of correlation and linear regression. His work with Galton's data helped to establish *probability distributions*, which are the statistical bedrock of modern psychometric theory. Actual clinical measurement of abilities and the statistical methods developed to describe these measurements were the starting place for the burgeoning field of psychometrics (Porter, 2004).

Wilhelm Wundt (1832–1920) is often credited with establishing the first laboratory of psychology at the University of Leipzig. The range and scope of his writings was immense, and his work is regarded as establishing psychology as a separate and distinct field of inquiry. From a distance, Wundt's approach to the study of psychology was less practically oriented than that of Galton. Wundt was known for developing the technique of introspection, which he believed was an important method for understanding basic psychological processes. More generally, Wundt's laboratory was associated with the development of experimental and physiological psychology, as well as a range of statistical techniques to describe and quantify abilities that were the focus of the new field of psychology. Wundt's student Charles Spearman (1863–1945) is widely known for developing *factor analysis* and for his discovery of the general factor ("g"), in cognitive or intellectual abilities. These contributions were important milestones in the development of tasks and theories that would form the basis of early intelligence tests (Boring, 1950).

Early developmental psychologists were also interested in the assessment of abilities, though their focus was more utilitarian than that of the psychometricians. Alfred Binet (1857–1911) is credited with producing the first usable measure of intellectual abilities. Binet earned his law degree in 1878, but was intrigued with education and intelligence and essentially became a self-taught psychologist. He spent several years in the 1880s working with Charcot at the Salpetriere, but a lack of success with studies on hypnosis and the birth of his daughters is said to have shifted Binet's focus to intellectual development. He took a position at the Sorbonne's Laboratory of Experimental Psychology in the early 1890s and eventually became its director. His work with his student Theodore Simon (1872–1961) resulted in what is referred to as the Binet–Simon scale, the first usable intelligence test. The test was developed for the purposes of identifying students with intellectual limitations, and it consisted of a number of tasks that were thought to be representative of a typical child's abilities at a specific age (Fancher, 1998).

The simplistic notion of a *mental age* was something that Binet cautioned against (Siegler, 1992), though it obviously had considerable traction and influence as others began to develop intelligence tests. The term *intelligence quotient* (IQ) was first proposed by German psychologist William Stern in 1912 and consisted of the basic formula mental age divided by chronological age. This method was abandoned long ago in favor of distribution-based statistical formulae for characterizing intellectual abilities. While statistical formulae and distribution parameters are centrally important in modern neuropsychological thinking, notions about cognitive development are also critical to understanding performance on neuropsychological test measures.

Swiss psychologist Jean Piaget (1896–1980) worked with Binet and Simon early in his career, though he was less interested in tests of intelligence than he was in the adaptive nature of intelligence and how that grew over time. Piaget's stages of intellectual development and his ideas about *assimilation* and *accommodation* are among the most influential ideas in education and child development. They have also influenced notions about how to assess cognitive abilities in children and re-emerged in neuropsychology as clinicians began to specialize in pediatric practice (Zigler & Gilman, 1998).

Intelligence Testing Foundations

With developmental psychologists paving the way with tests to assess intellectual skills, academics and clinicians with specific goals began to develop lengthier and better standardized measures of intelligence. Lewis Terman (1877–1956) was an American psychologist who began his career as a school principal and subsequently moved into academia. He was interested in assessing the ability of children and using this information to predict performance later in life. In 1916, at Stanford University, Terman adapted and standardized the Binet–Simon Scale for use with American subjects and called it the Stanford Revision of the Binet–Simon Scale—or Stanford–Binet, as it has been known for nearly one hundred years. Terman utilized Stern's simple quotient (IQ), multiplying the ratio by 100 to obtain the index score that, for better or worse, has become synonymous with "intelligence."

Like Terman, Henry Goddard (1866–1957) was also involved in education and was the first to translate the Binet–Simon Scale and distributed it widely throughout the United States. Goddard was involved in most of the large-scale efforts to develop tests for various classification purposes, including the Army Alpha and Beta tests for military recruits that were led by Robert Yerkes (1876–1956). The popularity of these tests was immense, and there was great hope that they could be used to classify individuals in a manner that would improve the fortunes of a young and ambitious country.

For these same reasons, misguided notions about eugenics and improving the lot of society would be held up as ideals that could be served by these powerful new tests. Throughout much of the twentieth century, spirited debates would be waged regarding what such tests could actually tell us and how they might be most appropriately utilized (Sternberg & Grigorenko, 1997). Early neuropsychologists would avoid much of this controversy by reverting to Binet's original purpose of using tests to identify preserved skills and limitations, in order to provide appropriate care and supervision of those with cognitive challenges. The most important and enduring legacy of these early test developers is the tests that they devised. Many subtests from the original Binet–Simon scale and the Army Alpha measures remain to a substantial degree in the latest versions of standardized intelligence measures and various neuropsychological tests (Boake, 2000).

The availability of increasingly well-standardized measures of mental abilities made assessment of wide-ranging clinical populations possible, and this development represented the beginnings of clinical neuropsychology as we know and practice it in the present day. Much of what was accomplished by these pioneers could be characterized as normative explorations. That is, test developers were cobbling together batteries of tests that were borrowed from earlier investigations and were finding out what worked and what did not. Two large-scale assessment efforts would galvanize the importance of mental testing in the United States and would also foreshadow the importance of considering the special needs and challenges of different clinical populations.

The first of these efforts involved the assessment of immigrants coming to Ellis Island in the early part of the twentieth century (Knox, 1914). The limitations of the earliest intelligence tests (most notably the Binet–Simon) became clear when non-English speaking and largely uneducated individuals were to be evaluated in some fashion. Boake (2000) suggests that Howard Knox may have been the first to use the term *performance tests* to describe measures that did not rely on comprehension of an unfamiliar language or extensive educational background. These progenitors of so-called culturally fair measures consisted mainly of puzzles, blocks, and form board tests that would presumably not require educational background or much language mediation. *Performance* scales would remain so-named through the third revisions of both the Wechsler child and adult intelligence scales (Wechsler, 1991; 1997). The important legacy of such measures was the realization that individuals needed to be assessed with adapted measures based on the group's limitations, and this would be particularly important when assessing clinical populations.

The second and perhaps most wide-ranging testing program in history involved the testing of recruits for the U.S. Army during World War I (Yerkes, 1921). Two primary group-administered measures were developed and were called Group Examination Alpha and Group Examination Beta. The Alpha was for recruits who spoke and read English, while the Beta was designed for use with individuals who were not proficient in English or who were illiterate. A good deal of the content for the Alpha was adapted from the Stanford–Binet. Group administration was facilitated by using a multiple choice format, objective scoring techniques, and time limits. Yerkes (1921) estimated that over 1,700,000 recruits were given the Alpha and Beta examinations. David Wechsler (1896–1981) borrowed extensively from the Alpha and Beta tests in the original Wechsler Bellevue scale, essentially changing the items to an individual administration format. Thus, item content from Binet's original measure made its way into many future generations of intelligence tests and remains in current day measures. Boake (2000) provides an excellent review of the development of intelligence tests that is well beyond the scope of this chapter. However, the importance of these measures as tools used in neuropsychological assessment cannot be overstated.

Neuropsychological Assessment Foundations

The importance of (1) using measures that are appropriate to the limitations of an individual or group and (2) rigorous normative standardization are concepts that evolved from the substantial efforts of those developing intelligence tests. Those basic psychometric concepts continue to undergird contemporary neuropsychological thinking. Intelligence tests have evolved very slowly over the past century in terms of their content, and their inclusion in the modal neuropsychological evaluation is often to establish the stability of basic intellectual skills. More recent revisions of the Wechsler scales (Wechsler, 2003; 2008) have paid homage to neuropsychological theories with the addition of new subtests, and the jettisoning of indices (e.g., Verbal and Performance IQs) and subtests (e.g., Object Assembly, Picture Arrangement) that do not contribute to the underlying factor structure of the test as determined by the scientific literature. In contrast to the relatively invariant content of traditional intelligence tests, modern neuropsychological measures have developed to assess differences in cognitive functioning that are the result of underlying neurologic impairment or pathology. Unlike intelligence indices, which are often insensitive to changes hastened by brain impairment, neuropsychological tests are designed for the expressed purpose of identifying impairment that might not be readily apparent using basic ability measures.

Early neuropsychologists came to utilize psychological or mental tests to identify deficits in individuals afflicted by different forms of brain damage (Barr, 2008; Boake 2000). In the United States, Europe, and Russia psychologists worked with varied clinical populations, most prominently soldiers injured in wartime. Patients surviving head injuries comprised a major portion of this sample. Neuropsychologists were charged with assessing various patient groups, and they utilized tests drawn both from intelligence measures and psychophysical tasks from various experimental psychology laboratories. Barr (2008) summarizes the development of different approaches to neuropsychological assessment and points to the fact that these approaches have different philosophical roots. According to Barr (2008), Wilhelm Wundt and Jean-Martin Charcot were the early progenitors of the functionalist and Gestalt approaches that emerged in the early days of psychology.

In the early history of neuropsychology, a well-known proponent of the *functionalist approach* was Ward Halstead (1908–1968) from the University of Chicago. He developed a battery of measures for the purpose of assessing biological intelligence (Halstead, 1947). This battery would later be adapted by his student Ralph Reitan for clinical use and would come to be known as the *Halstead–Reitan Neuropsychological Test Battery (HRB)* (Reitan & Wolfson, 1985). Halstead's painstaking approach in selecting instruments was described by Reitan (1994), who explained that Halstead was not unappreciative of the importance of qualitative observation, but rather was interested in assuring the reliability of a method that did not rely on nuanced observational skills. The importance of the battery associated with Halstead's name cannot be underestimated in the development of today's clinical neuropsychology. It established the importance of a data-oriented approach that emphasized rigorous standardization and the scientific method, and arguably allowed the profession to be considered a science in the same realm as medicine.

In contrast to the data-based empiricism represented by the HRB, another school of thought emerged from the realm of clinical medicine (Lamberty, 2002). This approach attended to behaviors evident in the process of solving tasks set before patients and was more consonant with the *Gestalt approach* to psychology (Barr, 2008). Kurt Goldstein (1878–1965) was a German neurologist whose allegiance to the Gestalt school typified a more qualitative approach to understanding brain function and dysfunction. Performance on tests was still central to the assessment enterprise, but scores were regarded as having relatively limited value outside of the manner in which individuals performed tasks (Goldstein & Scheerer, 1941). In neuropsychology, Goldstein is often remembered for his suggestion that brain-injured patients suffered a loss of "abstract attitude," and that this was often related to damage to the frontal lobes (Goldstein, 1990). However, it was also true that abstraction was impaired in all manner of other psychopathologic states that were not clearly characterized by frontal dysfunction. Goldstein's broader interest in psychopathology and behavior was not reflective of neuropsychology's emerging obsession with structure and function relationships, though it was arguably a more realistic view.

Since the mid-twentieth century, many other neuropsychologists have approached the study of brain and behavior in a way that was more process oriented, including the Russian neuropsychologist Alexander Luria (1902–1977). Luria was well known for his painstaking qualitative description of patients' performance on clinically oriented measures (e.g., Luria, 1966). In more recent times, the *Boston Process approach* (e.g., Goodglass & Kaplan, 1979) emerged as a prominent qualitative approach to assessing patients that focused on the nature and quality of performance rather than test scores alone (Milberg, Hebben, & Kaplan, 2009). While the qualitative nature of these approaches was central, it would be erroneous to assert that standardization and use of scores were unimportant. A number of today's most widely used measures were developed from within the process model (e.g., Delis et al., 2000) and include huge standardization samples with excellent psychometric properties. This is an illustration of a general trend that acknowledges the importance of both rigorous standardization and understanding of the importance of qualitative features of performance.

Several prominent twentieth-century neuropsychologists like Hans-Lukas Teuber (1916–1977), Oliver Zangwill (1913–1987), and Arthur Benton (1909–2006) used established measures and developed their own tests to capture the unique features of the classical syndromes that they observed in their respective clinic settings. For example, tests developed in the

University of Iowa laboratory that bears Arthur Benton's name have long been associated with a "hypothesis testing" approach that is the foundation of the dominant approach to neuropsychological assessment in the present day (Tranel, 2009).

In his excellent summary of the development of neuropsychological test batteries, Barr (2008) points out the fact that neuropsychological test batteries over the years have typically shared many tests, and the tests employed were often developed for purposes that did not originally involve the assessment of brain functioning. Indeed, recent practice surveys (Sweet, Nelson, & Moberg, 2006; Sweet et al., 2011) suggest that neuropsychologists have moved away from a standardized battery and toward a *flexible battery approach*—perhaps suggesting that the benefits of both traditions and approaches are being utilized. However, this is not necessarily the case and many have cautioned against accepting such trends without a critical appraisal of why our assessments are comprised of the measures they are (Russell, 1997; Lamberty, 2002; Barr, 2008).

The field of clinical neuropsychology as a well-defined subspecialty of clinical psychology is grounded in the rich traditions of behavioral neurology, psychiatry, psychometric assessment, and statistics. The field has evolved dramatically over the last century, and the future will almost certainly involve development of novel measures marked perhaps by briefer assessments. As discussed later in this book, choices will be guided by the clinical and economic outcomes literature and neuropsychology should be well capable of doing the work that is needed to guide these decisions. How the field rises to this challenge is likely to have a lasting impact on neuropsychology practice into the foreseeable future.

TWO

Professional Practice of Clinical Neuropsychology

In chapter 1 we briefly reviewed the historical roots of clinical neuropsychology, emphasizing developments from the end of the nineteenth century through the mid- to later portions of the twentieth century. While the nature of neuropsychology practice has evolved in a steady manner, organizations associated with practitioners of clinical neuropsychology have been very active over the past 40 years.

As also noted in chapter 1, professional organizations tend to develop when a field of inquiry achieves a critical mass of people who share an identity based on their interests, duties, and sense of purpose. From within these ranks a profession's ideas about what constitutes a specialty begin to emerge and, in turn, there is increased need to communicate these ideas to the public. Ironically, practitioners of a specialty often seem to neglect these needs until such a time that the promulgation of standards and guidelines is forced upon them by outside sources. Issues that seem self-evident to those within the field are not necessarily understood or appreciated by those who utilize its services. Thus, the task of clarifying the product and its value eventually becomes a priority. Several different organizations have emerged since the 1960s and have influenced how the field, its subject matter, and the background of its practitioners are defined. This has been particularly true in clinical neuropsychology over the past 10 to 20 years (APA CRSPPP, 2010; Heilbronner, 2007; INS/Division 40, 1987; NAN, 2001).

What follows is a description of organizations and events that have been central to promoting the field and developing definitions and guidelines for clinical practice in clinical neuropsychology. Table 2.1 includes a

Table 2.1 **Historical Milestones in the Development of Definitions and Guidelines for the Profession of Clinical Neuropsychology**

1967: International Neuropsychological Society established
1976: INS Committee on Scientific and Professional Affairs established
1980: APA Division 40 — Clinical Neuropsychology established
1987: Reports of the INS/Division 40 Task Force on Education, Accreditation, and Credentialing offers guidelines for training programs (Appendix A) 1989: Division 40 approves Definition of a Clinical Neuropsychologist (Appendix B)
1996: Committee for the Recognition of Specialties and Proficiencies in Professional Psychology recognizes clinical neuropsychology as a specialty (Appendix C)
1997: Houston Conference on specialty education and training in clinical neuropsychology convenes and produces a model of specialty training in clinical neuropsychology (Appendix D)
2001: National Academy of Neuropsychology approves definition of a clinical neuropsychologist (Appendix E)
2007: American Academy of Clinical Neuropsychology publishes Practice Guidelines for Neuropsychological Assessment and Consultation (Appendix F)

summary of historical milestones in clinical neuropsychology that are discussed in the next several pages.

International Neuropsychological Society

The early history of the International Neuropsychological Society (INS) has been detailed in a number of articles and transcripts (Costa, 1976; Costa, 1998; Meier, 1992; Rourke & Murji, 2000). The INS was the first organization to support the research and clinical interests of those involved in the burgeoning field of neuropsychology. Initially, the group was diverse and identified more by interests in neuropsychology than by a shared title of neuropsychologist or a standardized training curriculum. In fact, the early membership was split roughly between psychologists and physicians (with a substantial proportion of physiological, as opposed to clinical, psychologists). Rourke and Murji (2000) noted that the focus of informal groups from the midwestern United States and the East Coast seemed to be 1) the definition of a clinical specialty and 2) development of a formal society, respectively. These fundamental interests would shape the INS as time passed and also seemed to serve as the impetus for development of other neuropsychology-oriented groups. As with many organizations, the early history of the INS was rocky and characterized by uncertainty regarding its ultimate focus and even the need for such a group. INS began informally in 1965 when individuals from around the United States convened in Minneapolis (Rourke & Murji, 2000) at a meeting hosted by Manfred Meier. This group subsequently met in other locations and typically in conjunction with the annual American Psychological Association (APA) conferences. By the early 1970s, INS had initiated its own meeting, which steadily gained in popularity. By the mid-1970s the INS was ensconced as the world's preeminent neuropsychology organization.

In 1976, the INS meeting in Toronto represented something of a turning point for the specialty of clinical neuropsychology in the United States. INS president Louis Costa noted that clinical training standards would be necessary to define a specialty area, but that the INS was not necessarily ideally positioned to undertake such efforts (Costa, 1976). In his address, Costa suggested that it was perhaps time to consider formation of a division of a clinical neuropsychology within the APA. In September of 1976, the INS Committee on Scientific and Professional Affairs was established. Among this group's goals were interaction with other professional societies, the development of standards for education and credentialing in neuropsychology practice, and accreditation of clinical neuropsychology programs. From within this group, the Task Force on Education, Accreditation, and Credentialing of Clinical Neuropsychologists emerged. It subsequently merged with APA Division 40 (upon its establishment in 1980) to form the INS/Division 40 Task Force on Education, Accreditation, and Credentialing. Several portions and iterations of this group's recommendations were published in newsletters, with the final draft being published in *The Clinical Neuropsychologist* (Reports of the INS/Division 40 Task Force on Education, Accreditation and Credentialing, 1987; see Appendix A).

It is noteworthy that this document made recommendations for 1) doctoral training programs, 2) internships, and 3) postdoctoral training, perhaps assuming that a new generation of doctoral level clinical neuropsychology training programs would emerge. Such a sequence would be different from a more typical track in which neuropsychologists came primarily from clinical psychology doctoral programs. Ten years later, the APA Committee for the Recognition of Specialties and Proficiencies in Professional Psychology (APA CRSPPP, 2010) and the *Houston Conference* (Hannay et al., 1998) acknowledged that the degree to which specialty competencies would be obtained from within the three levels of training (doctoral training, internship, postdoctoral fellowship) was variable and not necessarily something that needed to be specified (Hannay et al., 1998).

The seeds of specialty definitions and guidelines were sewn by early members of the INS, but the need for groups with a more specific focus on clinically related matters of training and credentialing was also apparent. In this climate, the division of Clinical Neuropsychology of the APA was established and quickly came to be one of APA's largest and most active divisions. The INS has remained a major force in education and inter-disciplinary organization of professional groups interested in brain-behavior relationships. The membership overlap between INS and other clinically oriented neuropsychology groups in the United States remains substantial.

American Psychological Association: Division 40 — Clinical Neuropsychology

As mentioned above, an APA division of Clinical Neuropsychology was first formally recommended in 1976 by the INS president, Louis Costa. Because INS represented diverse interests and was, at least by name, an international group, it was wary of leading the charge to establish educ-ational and training standards for North American neuropsychologists. Therefore, following the publication of the INS/Division 40 guidelines (Appendix A), INS distanced itself from these matters, presumably leaving such efforts to the newly formed Division 40 and other such groups to come. In 1989, the Division 40 Executive Committee published the more succinct "Definition of a Clinical Neuropsychologist" (Division 40, 1989; see Appendix B) that included references to peer review and a specific indication of the ABCN/ABPP diploma in clinical neuropsychology as evidence of competence. This would later become a major issue of conten-tion from those within different groups representing the field of clinical neuropsychology.

Puente and Marcotte (2000) provide a description of the early days of Division 40, as well as extensive background regarding the structure and function of its various offices and committees. Division 40 is currently the third largest division of the APA, with steady membership of over 4,000 from the early part of this decade through the present. The mission of Division 40, as outlined in its most recent bylaws,

> is to advance the specialty of clinical neuropsychology as a science and profession and as a means of enhancing human welfare. The Division addresses this mission by promoting excellence in clin-ical practice, scientific research, and professional education in the

public interest. The goals derived from this mission are to be achieved in cooperation with the American Psychological Association, other professional organizations, and the general public (http://www.div40.org/APA_Division_40_Bylaws_2005.pdf).

The fundamental structure and function of Division 40 has not changed appreciably since its inception. The focus of the division has always been oriented toward practicing neuropsychologists, though as its mission statement declares, science and professional education are also prominent foci of the division's efforts. A description of Division 40's various committees can be obtained by visiting their website and perusing the Committee Activities tab (http://www.div40.org/committee_activities.htm).

The division's advocacy and educational endeavors are subsumed under several committees and provide opportunities for members to become involved with these activities. While advocacy (particularly practice advocacy through the Practice Advisory Committee) has recently been a central focus of the division, there has been little movement regarding the definition of a clinical neuropsychologist, or practice guidelines, for the specialty of clinical neuropsychology since 1996. At that time, the Commission for the Recognition of Specialties and Proficiencies in Professional Psychology (APA CRSPPP; 2010; see Appendix C) recognized Clinical Neuropsychology as its first specialty area (11 specialties have since been recognized by CRSPPP). The public description of clinical neuropsychology states that "clinical neuropsychology is a specialty that applies principles of assessment and intervention based upon the scientific study of human behavior as it relates to normal and abnormal functioning of the central nervous system. The specialty is dedicated to enhancing the understanding of brain-behavior relationships and the application of such knowledge to human problems" (APA CRSPPP, 2010; see Appendix C).

The recognition of clinical neuropsychology as a specialty was the result of a great deal of effort of those involved in the early organizational history of clinical neuropsychology, but it arguably did little to provide structure or recommendations regarding what constituted a core set of education and training experiences. As such, the definition and parameters offered by CRSPPP were descriptive, but not prescriptive. One could not determine exactly how to secure the knowledge necessary to satisfy specialty status, only the fact that one was supposed to obtain it. Appendix C includes the full text of the public definition of the specialty of clinical neuropsychology (http://www.apa.org/ed/graduate/specialize/neuro.aspx).

In the intervening years, challenges to the Division 40 (1989) definition of a clinical neuropsychologist have been put forth. The Division 40 Executive Committee surveyed its membership in 2006 and considered a number of alternatives, including a revised definition. Division 40 leadership determined to take "a broader approach to provide guidance both to the public and the profession regarding the specialty of neuropsychology, through promulgation of guidelines for neuropsychology" (http://www.div40.org/def.html).[1] Around the time of this writing, Division 40 planned to put forth guidelines in the context of renewing their specialty designation with CRSPPP, though this did not occur based on information presented on the CRSPPP section of APA website.

Existing guidelines notwithstanding, the size of Division 40, its resources, and the backing of the APA obviously make it a major force in the field of clinical neuropsychology practice. The size of Division 40 also produces obstacles. Variability in the education, training, and experiential backgrounds of Division 40 membership is substantial. Individuals need only be members of the APA to qualify for Division 40 membership. In this context, promulgation of guidelines that might prove to be exclusive of some members will likely be challenging. Whatever the procedural challenges, it seems assured that any Division 40 guidelines will have an immediate and substantial impact on clinical and forensic neuropsychology practice.

On a grander scale, issues of board certification in professional psychology are even more complex and contentious than they are at the divisional level. Without relying on conjecture, it stands to reason that an organization the size of the APA (150,000 members) is compelled to serve the interests of members with hugely varied backgrounds and interests. In other words, APA is not simply a practice-based organization, and standing behind credentialing standards that would likely alienate a good portion of the membership does not seem likely. Further, support of specific non-APA organizations that certify competence is fraught with peril as members of various boards are broadly represented within the ranks of the APA and Division 40 membership. From within the APA, CRSPPP emerged as a vehicle for recognizing the existence of various specialty areas. However, CRSPPP does not as yet promulgate standards, examine applicants, or certify competence based on a peer review process.

---

[1] It is noteworthy that this approach was taken by the American Academy of Clinical Neuropsychology (AACN), which published guidelines in early 2007 (described later in this chapter).

The field of clinical neuropsychology will be vitally interested in guidelines produced by the APA and Division 40 should this ever come to fruition.

The Houston Conference

By the time that CRSPPP recognized clinical neuropsychology as a specialty area in 1996, the first set of standards recommending training and experiential standards for neuropsychologists had been in existence (in some form) for more than 10 years (Reports of the INS/Division 40 Task Force on Education, Accreditation and Credentialing, 1987). The CRSPPP recognition was an important milestone, but there continued to be a sense that specific specialty training standards were lacking. The Houston Conference on Specialty Education and Training in Clinical Neuropsychology (Houston Conference; Hannay et al., 1998), sought to fill that void. Participants of the Houston Conference (HC) were "a group of 37 clinical neuropsychologists [selected] to reflect diversity in practice settings, education and training models, specializations in the field of clinical neuropsychology, levels of seniority, culture, geographic location, and sex" (Appendix D). In addition, representatives from the National Academy of Neuropsychology (NAN), APA Division 40, the American Board of Clinical Neuropsychology, the American Academy of Clinical Neuropsychology, and the Association of Postdoctoral Programs in Clinical Neuropsychology attended as delegates from the sponsoring organizations. The group met for five days in early September, 1997 and their recommendations were published in a special issue of the Archives of Clinical Neuropsychology the following year (Hannay et al., 1998; see Appendix D).

The preamble for the conference stated that "there has been no widely recognized and accepted description of integrated education and training in the specialty of clinical neuropsychology. The aim of the Houston Conference was to advance an aspirational, integrated model of specialty training in clinical neuropsychology." At the time of its publication, the aspirational nature of the Houston Conference recommendations meant that no one would be bound to follow the model as part of an accreditation process, though the comprehensiveness of the recommendations provided a target for education and training programs.

Relative to the other published definitions and specialty guidelines, the HC document was far lengthier and more detailed. There are numerous sections in the policy statement covering definitions, knowledge base, skills, doctoral education, internship training, residency education and training, subspecialties, continuing education, diversity in education and training, and models of training. As such, questions left by previous definitions were at least partially answered. Education and training programs were provided with a model and individuals could identify specific goals to which they could aspire in order to refer to themselves as clinical neuropsychologists. The official policy statement for the Houston Conference is included in Appendix D.

Concerns about the Houston Conference emerged in the years following publication of the policy statement. Reitan et al. (2004) published a critique of the conference and included responses from 92 individuals from 158 "persons in Reitan's correspondence file." The main contention of the article was that the attendees of the Houston Conference were a highly self-selected group of individuals associated with university training programs, and that these individuals were not representative of rank and file practicing neuropsychologists or their experiences/concerns. As a result, general concerns about disenfranchisement of those already practicing neuropsychology and generations to come were held up as a major problem with the HC document. Other critiques have also been published (Ardila, 2002; Reynolds 2002), also mainly critical of the composition of the group that promulgated the HC guidelines and the impact on those currently practicing. It should be noted that all of the definitions and guidelines published have emphasized their aspirational nature. Clearly, individuals practicing neuropsychology at a given time may or may not meet criteria such as those proposed in the Houston Conference.

It has never been the case that any of the definitions or standards noted in this chapter were expected to be applied retroactively. Movements toward more demanding and restrictive standards are often viewed with wariness by those practicing in a particular field. In his Division 40 presidential address, Linas Bieliauskas criticized the notion that the welfare of the practitioner and "inclusiveness" should guide our choices about professional standards (Bieliauskas, 1999). Doing so would effectively place the needs and welfare of patients at a lower priority than that of practitioners. Medical practice in the United States evolved to its current state after contentious battles in the early part of the twentieth century (Stevens, 1978). These battles changed the training landscape in medicine from proprietary schools to a more university-based system—a movement that Bieliauskas (1999) argued is a mirror image of what seems to be happening in today's professional psychology landscape.

In the fall of 2002, the American Board of Clinical Neuropsychology (ABCN) determined that it would apply the HC guidelines for all applicants completing their doctoral degree after December 31, 2004. This recognition by the American Board of Professional Psychology's (ABPP) specialty board in clinical neuropsychology gave the Houston Conference guidelines a de facto stamp of approval as the prevailing education and training standards in the field. Of course, other organizations have not endorsed the HC standards in such a clear fashion. However, at the time of the publication of this volume an Interorganizational Summit on Education and Training (ISET) Steering Committee had been organized to examine the possibility of revisiting the recommendations made in the Houston Conference. Plans were under way for a survey of individuals from a number of neuropsychology membership organizations. Ultimately the group will determine whether there is a need for a Houston II conference. Regardless, at the time of this writing, the Houston Conference guidelines stand as the most comprehensive statement about training and education in clinical neuropsychology. To the extent that other guidelines might be promulgated, they will be judged against the HC model.

National Academy of Neuropsychology (NAN)

The National Academy of Neuropsychology was established in 1975 by a group of clinically oriented neuropsychologists. To date, there has not been a comprehensive published review of NAN's history in the neuropsychology literature, such as those provided for INS (Rourke & Murji, 2000) and Division 40 (Puente & Marcotte, 2000. According to its mission statement, NAN seeks "to advance neuropsychology as a science and health profession, to promote human welfare, and to generate and disseminate knowledge of brain-behavior relationships." The organization's primary vehicles for completing this mission have been a popular annual meeting featuring continuing education workshops and a scientific program (commencing in 1981), their official journal (*Archives of Clinical Neuropsychology*), and a charitable foundation that funds neuropsychologically oriented research and activities (the NAN Foundation). NAN has established a large membership (currently over 3,300) and has been involved in practice-related initiatives for many years.

The NAN website provides access to a number of position papers and documents to assist practitioners. As NAN's meeting grew in popularity and their membership base increased, the organization became increasingly involved in practice advocacy with the establishment of the Professional Affairs and Information Organization (now the Professional Affairs and Information Committee/PAIC). The NAN website contains many different resources for practitioners, including a number of position papers published through its Policy and Planning Committee (http://nanonline.org/NAN/ResearchPublications/PositionPapers.aspx). Of particular interest in this context, the NAN Policy and Planning Committee published the "Definition of a Clinical Neuropsychologist," described as expanding and modifying the definition offered by Division 40 (NAN, 2001; see Appendix E). The document is succinct and focuses on the minimal criteria considered necessary to practice the specialty of clinical neuropsychology. The criteria include:

1. a doctoral degree in psychology,

2. an internship,

3. two years of experience (one predoctoral and one postdoctoral), including supervision by a clinical neuropsychologist, and

4. a license to practice psychology.

The definition states that board certification in clinical neuropsychology is not required, but does provide further evidence of "advanced training, supervision, and applied fund of knowledge in clinical neuropsychology" (NAN, 2001).

There was further clarification in a footnote regarding individuals who trained and practiced prior to the offering of the NAN definition. Specifically, individuals who were practicing prior to 2001 and met the Division 40 criteria were considered to meet the NAN standards. Regardless of the stated purpose of the NAN definition, it did not provide guidance as to the nature of training experiences, but rather rough minimal criteria that were actually less exclusive than the Division 40 (1989) guidelines. Perhaps the greatest distinction between the two definitions was the fact that the NAN definition mentioned board certification only as "further evidence," whereas the Division 40 (1989) definition specified board certification through ABCN as the "clearest evidence of competence as a clinical neuropsychologist." It is also notable that the NAN definition made only passing reference to the CRSPPP recognition of clinical neuropsychology, and no mention of HC guidelines, which seem an unusual omission given that the NAN definition was published 4 years after the HC proceedings in the same journal.

As with Division 40, NAN is a large membership organization with great diversity in training backgrounds. The brevity of the 2001 definition likely related to many factors, though it clearly backed away from the notion that board certification was the "clearest evidence of competence" to practice in the field. This presumably related to the fact that most individuals identifying themselves as neuropsychologists were not board-certified, as well as the fact that there were two certifying boards with little membership overlap. As noted earlier, the Division 40 definition (1989) specified ABCN board certification as the clearest evidence of competence, and this view was challenged by those board-certified through the American Board of Professional Neuropsychology (ABN). During the time that the NAN definition was promulgated, their board of directors had strong representation from individuals who were board-certified through ABN. Once again, at the time of the publication of this book, it was rumored that NAN was working on standards of practice, but no mention of this was made on the NAN website or through their official journal.

Neuropsychology from the Consumer's Perspective

Issues of how we define ourselves and what we do professionally are closely intertwined. As the previous pages have indicated, it has been a challenge to produce a universally accepted definition of a clinical neuropsychologist, or training guidelines that are similarly widely accepted. Nevertheless, such definitions are important starting points for a young field. They presumably speak to issues of import such as subject matter, knowledge base, and expected background experiences. In the present day, clinical neuropsychology is a widely recognized practice area in which practitioners are able to use specific procedural codes for reimbursement purposes. In other words, clinical neuropsychology is an economically established reality. As such, consumers (patients, family members, various care providers, third-party payers) should be able to determine what to expect when they are referred for, or in some way partake in, the neuropsychological assessment process. The CRSPPP archival description of clinical neuropsychology provides some basic detail regarding populations served and the fact that specific procedures are employed. However, little detail is provided that would allow a clear and comprehensive understanding of what constitutes an appropriate neuropsychological evaluation.

The major neuropsychology groups (e.g., AACN, Division 40, NAN) have provided some information along these lines. Brochures and various white papers have been produced for the purpose of educating consumers about what kinds of services are available from clinical neuropsychologists. While these are helpful for patients and their families, insurance companies and others who reimburse for neuropsychology services are likely to want more of an evidence base to assure that funds are being used in a responsible and clinically expedient manner. The emergence of evidence-based practice in psychology (EBPP; APA, 2006) has been an important development, and it encourages empirically validated standards for clinical decision making. In the modern health care climate there are increasing expectations that practitioners can provide evidence of the worth of their services. If professional guilds are unable to marshal their resources in this way, the stability of their field is lessened and the likelihood that reimbursement for services will continue presumably diminishes.

Therefore, practice standards or guidelines are increasingly important as a means of communicating the purpose and worth of services provided. As mentioned at the outset of this chapter, if practitioners do not lead the efforts to define their practice area, others involved in the health care marketplace certainly will. This includes various health care service companies who provide advice that is presumably based on the extant scientific and clinical literature. Across the United States, battles are being fought regarding decisions made by health care insurers bolstered by reviews of the scientific literature by individuals who have little or no clinical practice experience. Such challenges provided the backdrop for efforts by the American Academy of Clinical Neuropsychology (AACN) in their efforts to produce practice guidelines for their members and neuropsychology practitioners in general.

THE AMERICAN BOARD OF CLINICAL NEUROPSYCHOLOGY (ABCN) AND AMERICAN ACADEMY OF CLINICAL NEUROPSYCHOLOGY (AACN)

The American Academy of Clinical Neuropsychology is the membership organization for individuals who are board-certified under the auspices of the American Board of Clinical Neuropsychology (ABCN), which is a member board of the American Board of Professional Psychology (ABPP). ABCN was incorporated in 1981 by individuals who comprised the INS/Division 40 Joint Task Force on Credentialing in Clinical Neuropsychology (Yeates & Bieliauskas, 2004). Despite their important early work in defining the specialty, there was no credential that distinguished an individual as a clinical neuropsychologist. ABCN was formed to provide such a credential. In 1983 a formal affiliation between ABCN and the American Board of Professional Psychology (ABPP) was established, making clinical neuropsychology ABPP's fifth recognized specialty (after clinical, counseling, industrial/organizational, and school psychology). In 1996 ABPP required its specialty boards to establish membership academies as legally distinct organizations that could participate in a broader range of education and advocacy activities. As a result, AACN was formed (Ivnik, Haaland, & Bieliauskas, 2000; Yeates & Bieliauskas, 2004).

AACN has been active in a wide range of education and advocacy activities since its inception. Particularly impressive movement in these activities began around 2003 when the academy established an annual conference and affiliated with the *Clinical Neuropsychologist* as its official journal (Lamberty, 2009; Sweet, 2008). At AACN's first annual conference in 2003, Robert Heilbronner proposed the establishment of a practice guidelines working group and the effort was endorsed by the AACN board of directors. The guidelines group produced a document that was the result of three years of effort, multiple reviews from the board of directors, and critiques from a group of senior reviewers (Heilbronner, 2007). The AACN Practice Guidelines document was "intended to serve as a guide for the practice of neuropsychological assessment and consultation and is designed to promote quality and consistency in neuropsychological evaluations" (p. 210).

The AACN Practice Guidelines document is significantly different from the documents described earlier in this chapter. They are broad in scope and focus on the nature of neuropsychological assessment and consultation. The guidelines provide a general framework for what is typically included in an assessment, from initial contact through the written report and subsequent feedback. There is no specific mention of individual tests, but rather a focus on the nature of the tests and the fact that there should be a scientific basis and ample validity studies supporting the use of all measures. Appendix E includes the reprinted text of the AACN Practice Guidelines, and the original paper is also available through the AACN website (http://www.theaacn.org/position_papers/AACNPractice_Guidelines.pdf).

At its annual meeting in 2009, AACN announced the formation of the AACN Foundation (AACNF), whose specific charge was to raise and distribute funds for the purpose of funding outcomes research in clinical neuropsychology. At the 2010 annual conference, AACNF announced it first grant awardees and sought to continue to raise funds for additional studies. The economic climate provided a considerable challenge as neuropsychologists struggled with declining reimbursement from Medicare and similar declines from health care insurers.

As mentioned earlier, circumstances in the practice world have provided a greater sense of urgency with respect to more universally endorsed practice guidelines. Whether these exigencies will facilitate cooperation between the important neuropsychology organizations and allow a coherent and meaningful set of guidelines to be established is yet to be determined. It is clear that clinical neuropsychology is a very highly organized specialty practice area with an impressive track record of efforts to define training standards and the nature of consultation and practice. At the time of the publication of this book, the *Clinical Neuropsychology Synarchy (CNS)* was gathering together a group of representatives from major membership organizations in clinical neuropsychology for this very purpose.

Problems Addressed by Clinical Neuropsychologists

Neuropsychologists have assumed a wide range of professional and clinical roles as the profession has matured (Lamberty, Courtney & Heilbronner, 2003). Early neuropsychologists typically operated in hospital settings conducting assessments with head trauma, stroke, and various neurosurgical patients. They served as diagnosticians, given their ability to determine brain impairment and to localize damage with accuracy equal to or better than the technologies of the day. Today, a wide range of increasingly sophisticated structural and functional imaging techniques have made the basic localization function of early neuropsychology considerably less relevant than it once was. Table 2.2 summarizes common problems for which neuropsychologists offer their services in modern neuropsychology practice. While the primary goal of assessing cognitive difficulties continues to be the most prominent and obvious reason for referral, other issues have gained prominence based on factors that go beyond the basic description of neuropsychology as the study of brain-behavior relationships.

Neuropsychologists possess skills in assessing and understanding cognitive and emotional difficulties that allow them to assist with referring for and treating a range of clinical concerns that go beyond difficulties with

Table 2.2 **Common Problems Addressed by Clinical Neuropsychologists**

1. Assessing the neuropsychological abilities of individuals with reported difficulties in cognitive functioning.

2. Characterizing functioning in complex cases involving medical and neuropsychiatric co-morbidities.

3. Assisting treatment teams or primary care providers with recommendations regarding most effective treatment approaches.

4. Conducting independent assessments in medico-legal contexts to assist triers of fact in making determinations about disability or damages.

5. Providing therapy and/or rehabilitation services to individuals with neuropsychological impairment.

6. Consulting with other professionals and scientists regarding eliciting or assessing specific cognitive functions.

cognitive functioning. For example, understanding the complex interplay between cognitive and psychological/emotional factors continues to be a major challenge for primary care personnel and those treating patients with complex presentations (Lamberty, 2007. This is also true in the rehabilitation context, where neuropsychologist and rehabilitation psychologists have long worked together with overlapping duties but slightly different goals (Wilson, 2009). The neuropsychologist's input in forensic matters has become increasingly courted, and there has been an explosion in work looking at symptom validity or malingering assessment (e.g., Sweet, 1999; Larrabee, 2005). It is interesting to note that much of the opportunity in clinical neuropsychology appears to relate to the more psychological side of the enterprise—that is, understanding the emotional concomitants of various disorders, assessing motivation, and providing therapeutic consultation and services have become the areas in which the services of neuropsychologists are most valued. This is something of a departure from the strictly assessment-oriented approach that came into prominence in neuropsychology practice in the late part of the last century. Thus, instead of assessment and diagnosis being the primary end-product of neuropsychological practice, there is now greater interest in how assessments inform subsequent disposition and treatment of referred patients. This includes not only treatment of cognitive difficulties, but encompasses general adjustment, psychological health, and management in general medical or primary care contexts.

It has long been recognized that the combination of imaging techniques and neuropsychological assessment can provide insights that were simply not possible in the past (Division 40, 2004). For some time, it has been suggested that the future of neuropsychology will encompass just such a hybrid practice involving neuroradiology and neuropsychology. Of course, these suggestions typically come from those most intimately involved in imaging science. The extent to which imaging science and neuropsychology merge to form a new neuropsychology is not clear and will doubtless be impacted by views in the health care profession about the value of such practices.

Populations Served by Clinical Neuropsychologists

A number of volumes have highlighted the broad range of populations served by clinical neuropsychologists (Morgan & Ricker, 2008; Grant & Adams, 2009; Lezak et al., 2004). Over time, the number of diagnoses and disorders for which there exists substantial neuropsychological data has markedly increased. It is certainly not the case that all neuropsychologists see such a range of diagnoses, but the availability of neuropsychological services and other professions' familiarity with neuropsychology increase the likelihood that neuropsychologists will be consulted in cases in which there are concerns with cognitive difficulties. Further, the expansion of pediatric neuropsychology over the past 20 or more years has increased the range and number of referral sources to the realm of pediatric practice (Yeates, et al., 2010).

Early practitioners in neuropsychology focused on neurological and neurosurgical populations including stroke and traumatic brain injury (e.g., Benton, 2000), though it became clear that neuropsychologists had a great deal to offer other patients and practitioners; the scope of neuropsychology practice broadened considerably from the 1980s through the present day (Grant & Adams, 2009; Morgan & Ricker, 2008). Thus, in addition to neurologically oriented diagnoses, it has become more common for patients with neuropsychiatric diagnoses such as bipolar disorder and posttraumatic stress disorder to be referred for neuropsychological evaluation. Further, referrals from primary care settings often involve patients with pain and somatoform diagnoses that include prominent concerns about cognitive difficulties (Lamberty, 2007. In reality, any patient with concerns about cognitive functioning is a potential referral for neuropsychological evaluation. In many ways, the skill of neuro-psychologists in a range of assessment techniques has made the referral of patients with a wide range of concerns a natural and broad base for neuropsychology practice. Some neuropsychologists believe that patients with issues that are primarily psychiatric in nature are not appropriate, though most would agree that there is value in distinguishing between cognitive difficulties that are related to neurologic versus functional causes.

In terms of most common populations seen for neuropsychological evaluation, recent surveys by Sweet and colleagues (Sweet, Nelson, & Moberg, 2006; Sweet et al., 2011) listed the five most common diagnoses seen by pediatric and adult practitioners, and those who treated "mixed" sets of patients.

- Common to all groups was traumatic brain injury, true to the field's history.
- Learning disability and attention deficit disorders were commonly seen across all groups of practitioners.
- Aging related dementias were common to adult and mixed practitioners.

- Seizure disorders were among the most commonly seen patients for pediatric neuropsychologists, though the frequency of seizure disorder cases declined in the most recent survey for adult and mixed practitioners (Sweet et al., 2011).
- Mood disorder patients are seen less frequently in the most recent survey, apparently being replaced by general medical and neurological conditions in adult and mixed practices.

Pediatric practitioners reported the same top five conditions, with only slight changes in order. Not surprisingly, pervasive developmental disorders are seen frequently by pediatric neuropsychologists, but not by other neuropsychologists (Sweet, Nelson, & Moberg, 2006; Sweet et al., 2011). As with many clinical matters, the health care marketplace will determine whether or how these patterns will change over time.

Subspecialization in Clinical Neuropsychology

Specialization in any field is typically based on several factors. Individual researchers and clinicians focus their efforts on specific populations or disorders as a matter of interest and expediency. Like-minded colleagues see value in convening to discuss cases and expound upon theories that develop in their practices. Within larger groups or specialties, interest groups are born and journals emerge to offer opportunities to specialists who may believe that their specialty is less interested or welcoming than would be ideal. Practically speaking, whether there is a need for subspecialization is often an economically determined matter. Payors (insurance companies and other vendors) often seek to assure the competence of providers beyond basic requirements for licensure. Similarly, medical staff organizations look for ways to determine that practitioners have been judged to be competent by their peers. In the medical field, this has translated into third-party organizations *requiring* board certification through a specialty board of the American Board of Medical Specialties (ABMS), which currently has 24 approved such boards.

Each ABMS board has numerous subspecialty designations that seek to distinguish providers as experts in more specific areas of practice. As an example, the American Board of Psychiatry and Neurology (ABPN) currently has 12 subspecialties, some requiring board certification in neurology, some in psychiatry, and some requiring special certification in child neurology (http://www.abpn.com/cert_subspecialties.htm). While the goal of subspecialization would appear to be further identification of individuals with specialty expertise, the extent to which these designations are deemed useful by payors or the public is difficult to determine. Nevertheless, subspecialty groups come into being and enjoy varying degrees of success by virtue of their ability to convince colleagues or the public of the importance of recognizing the subspecialty. The viability of recognizing specialties and subspecialties is ultimately an economic matter. If there are not enough dues-paying members, or enough third-party recognition, subspecialties, no matter how well reasoned or intended, will likely die on the vine. The larger board structure can allow such groups to exist, even if it is clear that there is an essential lack of vitality or interest in the area.

In clinical neuropsychology there are groups of individuals who have specially developed skills in areas that go beyond the general requirements needed for board certification. Most notably, pediatric neuropsychology has been a significant area of inquiry and practice for many years (Yeates, et al., 2010), and a substantial subset of neuropsychologists certified by the American Board of Clinical Neuropsychology identify themselves as having expertise in pediatric neuropsychology. The Pediatric Neuropsychology Special Interest Group (PNSIG) was formed by the ABCN in order to more thoroughly study the potential need for subspecialization. The PNSIG first met in June of 2009 at the AACN annual conference in San Diego, and is giving the issue of subspecialization greater and ongoing consideration. Other subspecialty possibilities exist, such as geriatric neuropsychology and forensic neuropsychology, but efforts in these areas have not been as active or organized as the efforts behind a pediatric subspecialty. Time and perceived need will likely determine if and when there will be formalized subspecialties in clinical neuropsychology.

PART II

Functional Competency—
Assessment

THREE

Assessment Strategies

For the purposes of this chapter we will forgo a lengthy description of the development of modern assessment approaches in clinical neuropsychology in favor of a more descriptive and functional approach. In chapter 1, it was pointed out that neuropsychology emerged broadly from traditions of clinical medicine and psychometrics. These traditions roughly equate to the proverbial art and science that all clinical fields claim as essential parts of their profession. The success of modern medicine is arguably based on the ability of a clinician to adroitly merge these two traditions. Given individuals may appreciate scientific verity or clinical art to a greater or lesser extent when they consider what is important in selecting a doctor. Nonetheless, it is usually the case that the best doctors or providers are well-versed in the scientific background of their fields *and* skilled in applying that knowledge to the individual patient. Critics and commentators in many fields are wary that such dichotomies are short-sighted and illusory, not unlike debates about the separateness of mind and body (Lamberty, 2007). We will not attempt to make a determination about which tradition is more compelling, though we acknowledge that historically dominant approaches in clinical neuropsychology might be said to fall to a greater or lesser extent on either side of an "art versus science" dividing line.

Table 3.1 lists a number of different descriptors that are often applied to approaches and philosophies in clinical neuropsychology. The list is meant as a point of reference, as opposed to being a clear-cut way of characterizing elements of knowledge and practice. In neuropsychology, the empirical underpinnings of all approaches are ultimately viewed as critical regardless of whether an approach appears to be more artful or scientific.

Table 3.1 **Dichotomies Used in Clinical Neuropsychology**

Art	Science
Qualitative	Quantitative
Descriptive	Actuarial
Idiographic	Nomothetic
Cognitivism	Behaviorism
Process	Achievement
Process Approach	Fixed Battery

Throughout this text we will refer to these distinctions when describing the practice of clinical neuropsychology.

Barr (2008) provides a complementary treatment of these broad distinctions when describing the development of various neuropsychological test batteries in the twentieth century. He argues that the heavily *quantitative* tradition espoused by Halstead found its roots in the work of Wundt, who emphasized the scientific study of mental activities. In contrast, Charcot's views were arguably more person-centered and aligned with the views of Gestalt psychology, which was concerned with the whole as compared to the parts. Such *qualitative* views provided a foundation for various process-oriented approaches that focused on understanding patients and presentations in a more holistic way. In the last 20 to 30 years of the twentieth century there were two dominant approaches in clinical neuropsychology that have been broadly referred to as fixed battery (Reitan & Wolfson, 2009) and process (Milberg, Hebben, & Kaplan, 2009) approaches.

Many authors have described theoretical views of cognitive functioning and corresponding ways of evoking or characterizing these abilities (Barr, 2008; Goldstein & Incagnoli, 1997; Milberg, Hebben & Kaplan, 2009; Reitan & Wolfson, 2009; Smith, Ivnik, & Lucas, 2008; Tranel, 2009). Despite the fact that various approaches to assessing brain function differ markedly in how they conceptualize neuropsychological abilities, the actual tests used by those espousing different theoretical models have typically been very similar (Barr, 2008; Smith, Ivnik, & Lucas, 2008). Therefore, regardless of whether a neuropsychologist is more interested in the quality of the normative base behind a test or the manner in which the task is approached by the patient, the tests used are often largely the same. In this context, it may not be surprising that increasingly fewer neuropsychologists characterize their approach to assessment as being dictated by a fixed battery, or a hypothesis testing/process approach (Sweet, Nelson, & Moberg, 2006; Sweet et al., 2011).

In fact, over the past 20 years, there has been steady movement toward more flexible assessment approaches, to the extent that some familiar approaches have essentially become anachronistic (Sweet, Moberg & Suchy, 2000; Sweet, Nelson, & Moberg, 2006; Sweet et al., 2011). It is certainly not the case that approaches emerging in the latter half of the twentieth century lack merit or heuristic value, but rather that neuropsychological science has advanced to a point where the empirical support and clinical utility of certain measures cannot be ignored. This general trend may also be an indication that the benefits of both kinds of approaches have likely become apparent to a wider range of practicing neuropsychologists. This has resulted in a clinical landscape that is comprised of a majority of practitioners conducting evaluations using *flexible batteries* that select measures originating from a number of different traditions (Sweet, Moberg, & Suchy, 2000; Sweet, Nelson, & Moberg, 2006; Sweet et al., 2011).

Standardized Batteries in Clinical Neuropsychology

In the early developmental stages of what came to be known as the Halstead Reitan Neuropsychological Test Battery (HRB), Reitan noted that he and Halstead were both appreciative of nuances in the clinical presentation of individual patients and the fact that such observations could be clinically useful (Reitan, 1994). Nevertheless, in order to develop a method that was rigorously standardized and reproducible, it was determined that an invariant and empirical approach was needed. Differences in the observational skills of examiners could not be allowed to influence the data collected. Halstead sorted through dozens of measures before selecting ten that would eventually be included in his work on "biological intelligence" (Halstead, 1947; Reitan & Wolfson, 2009). The measures were chosen to compare normal and brain-damaged subjects and the tests were administered as a group or battery. Reitan further modified the battery that would eventually also bear his name, excluding three of Halstead's original 10 tests and adding several that he found to optimally discriminate between normal and brain-damaged subjects (Reitan & Wolfson, 2009). Table 3.2 lists the measures that comprise the HRB in its current form.

It is clear that this rigorous empirical approach to characterizing patients' cognitive functioning was a boon to the practice of clinical

Table 3.2 **Tests of the Halstead Reitan Neuropsychological Test Battery (HRB)**

Halstead category test

Tactual performance test (TPT)

Trail making test

Seashore rhythm test

Speech-sounds perception test

Finger oscillation test

Grip strength (hand dynamometer)

Sensory perceptual examination

Aphasia screening test

Wechsler Adult Intelligence Scale

Minnesota Multiphasic Personality Inventory

neuropsychology. Neuropsychological evaluation was and is highly regarded as a valid and reliable clinical service, in no small part because of the influence of the HRB. The strength of the efforts behind the establishment of the HRB and the resulting mountain of data generated in studying its properties provided a guide for researchers and clinicians through the twentieth century.

Despite the fact that the nature of what neuropsychologists are being asked to do has evolved considerably over the past 30 to 40 years, the HRB seemed to provide an irresistible road map for neuropsychology. Studies on the battery and its various components have continued into the twenty-first century and proponents continue to suggest that only the HRB has known validity as a battery—which is something a number of authors have stated that flexible batteries cannot claim (Reitan & Wolfson, 2009; Russell, 2009). Few neuropsychologists would dispute the fact that the purpose of neuropsychological assessment has moved beyond basic determinations of whether or not an individual is "brain-damaged." On this point Rohling, Williamson, Miller, & Adams, (2003) commented, "the question of 'Is there brain damage?' is either too simplistic or simply irrelevant."

The assertion that the HRB was the only validated, comprehensive neuropsychological battery resulted in efforts to make comparisons between the HRB and more flexible approaches to assessment. Several recent studies have compared the HRB to different standardized measures such as the Wechsler Adult Intelligence Scale (WAIS) and to flexible batteries, with results comparable to or better than the HRB impairment index (HII) and the general neuropsychological deficit scale (GNDS) on the basic matter of determining the presence or absence of brain damage (Larrabee, Millis, & Meyers, 2008; Loring & Larrabee, 2006; Rohling, Williamson, Miller, & Adams, 2003). Concerns regarding being tethered to a lengthy battery or measures that do not assess specific abilities of interest have frequently been expressed, and today's modal practitioner appears to have determined that a battery approach is no longer practical or even ideal (Sweet, Moberg, & Nelson, 2006; Sweet et al., 2011). From the outset, one of the primary concerns about the HRB was the amount of time taken to administer the battery. The entire battery including WAIS and MMPI typically takes anywhere from five to seven hours depending upon the patient and his or her limitations, not including supplementary measures of memory and other specific cognitive abilities.

Another battery approach gained prominence in the late 1970s which was based on the work of Luria and his methods as described by Christensen (1975). The ubiquity of the HRB in clinical and research practices provided a framework for the Luria Nebraska Neuropsychological Battery (Golden, Hammeke, & Purisch, 1978) in the sense that there was a general expectation that neuropsychological evaluations should be packaged as a standard set of tests that are normed together. There was no small irony in the attempt to quantify Luria's methods, though similar efforts characterized the eventual standardization of methods from the Boston Process Approach, as described in the next section. Thus, while the HRB provided a sound empirical basis for neuropsychological assessment, innovators like Edith Kaplan persisted in extending and quantifying the largely qualitative early approaches of Goldstein, Luria, and others. As time passed, the importance of both ends of the spectra noted in Table 3.1 were given their due.

The Boston Process Approach

In contrast to the highly empirical approach represented by the HRB, the Boston Process Approach (BPA) evolved as a set of methods that attended to underlying cognitive processes, rather than a strict adherence to the data generated by assessments of patients with brain damage and normal controls. In the BPA, the subtleties of behavior in individuals are closely scrutinized as a means of understanding problems with cognition (Milberg,

Hebben, & Kaplan, 2009). The developers of the BPA were interested in clinical questions that went beyond the determination of brain damage. Such questions involved characterizing spared and impaired abilities, approaches taken to solving basic and complex problems, and assisting with rehabilitation/treatment planning. The complexity of the methods employed and the huge variability in observed patient behavior were cited as evidence of the impracticality of the BPA for routine clinical practice. As noted in the previous section, concerns about variability in an individual's administration and observational skills were central to the appeal of fixed batteries. Eventually, however, the techniques and measures comprising the BPA came to be standardized, both in terms of methods and collection of normative data.

Examples of measures that were adapted by Edith Kaplan and colleagues in the BPA tradition are the WAIS-R as a Neuropsychological Instrument (Kaplan et al., 1991), the Kaplan-Baycrest Neurocognitive Assessment (Leach et al., 2000), and the California Verbal Learning Test (Delis et al., 2000). All of these measures are based on well-known and commonly utilized tests of cognitive functioning. Efforts were generally made to allow for the standard administration of tasks, with process-oriented procedures being added on to obtain additional information. These adaptations typically involved strategies used in clinical settings such as testing limits, cueing, and providing multiple choice formats to allow for the assessment of a broader range of behaviors than would typically be assessed by the original tests alone. On perceptual measures, close attention to the manner in which patients handled stimulus materials, performed constructional tasks, and the nature of visuospatial errors were all noted and recorded.

Throughout the mid-1980s and 1990s interest in process-oriented adaptations was high and increased efforts were made to collect normative data for the modified measures, as well as to publish and distribute them to a wider audience of neuropsychologists. The California Verbal Learning Test–II (Delis et al., 2000) is among the most commonly used memory measures in clinical practice today, and this probably relates to the extensive normative efforts behind it as much as the process-oriented indices available with the test. As with most measures in current use, the normative efforts applied to process-oriented tests was an essential component in their increased acceptance and use by neuropsychologists. Regardless of the philosophy behind neuropsychological assessment measures, the importance of a sound empirical foundation has been underscored in general clinical practice and in the forensic realm. This tradition is likely to bolster the place of neuropsychological assessment well into the future (Lamberty, 2002).

Flexible Batteries/Approaches in Clinical Neuropsychology

The previous sections described the developmental process associated with different approaches to assessment in the practice of clinical neuropsychology. Empiricism and underlying theoretical models of cognitive functioning are both important, but the exigencies of clinical practice call for measures that span the descriptive spectrum *and* provide a solid normative underpinning.

In this context, what has come to be known as the *flexible battery approach* makes use of various tests that may be administered according to the individual patient's needs, but that typically include a core set of frequently administered measures (e.g., select subtests from the WAIS-III/IV). In slight contrast, the flexible approach consists of a wide variety of tests that may be administered to suit the individual patient's needs, and does not include a core set of measures that is uniformly administered.

Both the BPA (Milberg, Hebben, & Kaplan, 2009) and the Iowa-Benton School of Neuropsychological Assessment (Tranel, 2009) have been perceived as espousing flexible approaches, as they emerged from rich clinical traditions that involved highly varied interview approaches based on individual patient presentations. Many early neuropsychologists such as Ward Halstead, Arthur Benton, Harold Goodglass, and Edith Kaplan learned much by observing neurologists and psychiatrists with widely varying backgrounds. They gained an appreciation for the nuances of individual presentations, which provided important perspectives that shaped their approaches to assessment.

In reality, the BPA and Benton approaches evolved in a manner that distinguished them as flexible batteries rather than flexible approaches (Milberg, Hebben, & Kaplan, 2009; Tranel, 2009). That is, over time it was apparent that having a small number of core measures administered to most every patient was advantageous and allowed for direct comparisons across important domains of cognitive functioning. It would appear that what has been learned through these esteemed traditions has translated to typical clinical practice (Heilbronner, 2007). Even more functionally, recent survey data suggest that since 1989, standardized and flexible approaches have waned dramatically (Sweet, Nelson, & Moberg, 2006; Sweet et al., 2011), while the flexible battery approach has become relatively commonplace for most clinical neuropsychologists (79% of survey respondents endorse this approach as their usual practice in the most recent survey; Sweet et al., 2011).

Therefore, in most instances test selection is likely to depend upon a specific referral question. For example, with a patient referred for neuropsychological evaluation of possible dementia, the clinician is likely to administer a number of learning/memory tasks as well as select measures from other cognitive domains to allow for formal diagnosis of dementia according to DSM-IV-TR (which requires evidence of impairment in memory function as well as at least one other cognitive domain). In the final section of this chapter (see Table 3.3), we list a number of different measures of neuropsychological functioning in current use. The list is by no means exhaustive, but focuses on widely used and well standardized/validated measures.

Table 3.3 **Select Measures of Neuropsychological Functioning Categorized by Cognitive Domain**

COGNITIVE DOMAIN	EXAMPLE MEASURES
Overall Cognitive Function/Brief Screening Measures	Dementia Rating Scale–2 (DRS-2; Jurica et al., 2001)
	Mini-Mental Status Examination (MMSE; Folstein et al., 1975)
	NEPSY: A Developmental Neuropsychological Assessment (Korkman et al., 1998)
	Repeatable Battery for the Assessment of Neuropsychological Status (RBANS; Randolph, 1998)
Intellectual Functioning	Wechsler Adult Intelligence Scale–3rd Edition (WAIS-III; Wechsler, 1997)
	Wechsler Adult Intelligence Scale–4th Edition (WAIS-IV; Wechsler, 2008)
	Wechsler Intelligence Scale for Children–4th Edition (WISC-IV; Wechsler, 2003)
	Stanford–Binet–Fifth Edition (SB5; Roid, 2003)
Academic Achievement	Wechsler Individual Achievement Test–2nd Edition (WIAT-II; Psychological Corp, 2002)
	Wide Range Achievement Test–Fourth Edition (WRAT-IV; Wilkinson & Robertson, 2006)
	Woodcock-Johnson III Tests of Achievement (WJ-III; McGrew & Woodcock, 2001)
Attention/Concentration	Brief test of Attention (BTA; Schretlen, 1997)
	Paced Auditory Serial Addition Test (PASAT; Gronwall, 1977)

Table 3.3: **(Continued)**

COGNITIVE DOMAIN	EXAMPLE MEASURES
	Conner's Continuous Performance Test–2nd Edition (CPT-II; Conners & MHS Staff, 2000)
Speech/Language	Boston Diagnostic Aphasia Examination–3rd Edition (BDAE-3; Goodglass et al., 2001)
	Boston Naming Test–2nd Edition (BNT-2; Kaplan et al., 2001)
	Controlled Oral Word Association Test (COWAT; Gladsjo et al., 1999)
	Multilingual Aphasia Examination–3rd edition (MAE-3; Benton et al., 1994)
Visual-Spatial Functions	Executive Clock Drawing Task (CLOX; Royall et al., 1998)
	Hooper Visual Organization Test (HVOT; Hooper, 1958)
	Judgment of Line Orientation (JLO; Benton et al., 1994)
Executive Functioning	Booklet Category Test (BCT; Reitan & Wolfson, 1995)
	Delis-Kaplan Executive Function Battery (D-KEFS; Delis et al., 2001)
	Ruff Figural Fluency Test (Ruff; 1996, 1998)
	Stroop Color Word Test (Golden; 1978)
	Trail Making Test (TMT, Reitan; 1955)
	Wisconsin Card Sorting Test (WCST; Heaton et al., 1993)
Learning/Memory	Brief Visuospatial Memory Test–Revised (BVMT-R; Benedict, 1997)
	California Verbal Learning Test–2nd Edition (CVLT-II; Delis et al., 2000)
	Children's Memory Scale (CMS; Cohen, 1997)
	Hopkins Verbal Learning Test–Revised (HVLT-R; Brandt & Benedict, 2001)
	Rey Auditory Verbal Learning Test (RAVLT; Strauss, Sherman, & Spreen, 2006)
	Rey-Osterrieth Complex Figure Test (Meyers & Meyers, 1995)
	Wechsler Memory Scale–3rd Edition (WMS-III; Wechsler, 1997)
	Wechsler Memory Scale–4th Edition (WMS-IV; Wechsler, 2008)
Sensory & Motor Functioning	Finger Tapping (Heaton et al., 2004)
	Grooved Pegboard (Heaton et al., 2004)
	Grip Strength (Heaton et al., 2004)

(Continued)

Table 3.3: **Select Measures of Neuropsychological Functioning Categorized by Cognitive Domain (*Continued*)**

COGNITIVE DOMAIN	EXAMPLE MEASURES
Symptom Validity/Effort	
Symptom Validity Tests (SVTs)	**Symptom Validity Indices ("embedded" measures)**
Forced Choice	*Orientation*
Word Memory Test (WMT, Green, 2003)	WMS-R: Info/Orient (Suchy & Sweet, 2000)
Test of Memory Malingering (TOMM, Tombaugh, 1996)	*Attention/Concentration*
Victoria Symptom Validity Test (VSVT, Slick et al., 1996)	WAIS-III Digit Span (Greiffenstein et al., 1994)
Computerized Assessment of Response Bias	*Intellectual*
(CARB, Green & Iverson, 2001)	WAIS-R/WAIS-III (Mittenberg et al., 2001)
Portland Digit Recognition Test	*Language*
(PDRT, Binder & Kelly, 1996)	COWAT (Demakis, 1999)
	Visual-Spatial
Non-Forced choice	Rey-Osterrieth (Lu et al., 2003)
Rey-15 & Recognition (Boone et al., 2002)	*Executive*
Dot Counting Test (Boone et al., 2001)	WCST (King et al., 2002)
Rey Word Recognition Test (Nitch et al., 2006)	BCT (Sweet & King, 2002)
b-Test (Boone et al., 2000)	Stroop (Lu et al., 2004)
	Learning/Memory
	CVLT/CVLT-II (Sweet et al., 2000)
	RAVLT (Boone et al., 2005)
	Motor
	Finger Tapping (Arnold et al., 2005)
	Grip Strength (Greiffenstein et al., 1996)
	Gladsjo et al., 1999

Commonly Employed Instruments in Clinical Neuropsychology

Chapter 4 will present a contemporary model of *case conceptualization* that is influenced by the early schools of thought reviewed in this chapter. As mentioned earlier, most neuropsychologists employ tests that did not necessarily emerge from one or another school of thought, but rather came to be utilized in different ways by neuropsychologists of different theoretical orientations. Table 3.3 provides a list of instruments in common use in the United States.

At the present time, there are numerous well-standardized and commercially available measures offered for use. The success of neuropsychology as a clinical field has resulted in a proliferation of tests offered by vendors, though many frequently used tests emerge from the scientific and clinical literature and remain in the public domain. Clearly, rigorously standardized measures have become the norm in the field, though this does not negate the potential value of new and unique measures and their subsequent development. Further, norms are in need of regular updating and this is often provided by the peer-reviewed literature as well. Neuropsychological assessment has not typically been prone to fads, and occasional surveys provide information about those measures that are in regular use (Butler, Retzlaff, & Vanderploeg, 1991; Camara, Nathan, & Puente, 2000; Rabin, Barr, & Burton, 2005). The focus of these surveys has been slightly different depending upon the stated purpose, and not all are strictly oriented to neuropsychological evaluation. Finally, the Buros Mental Measurement Yearbook has been in yearly print since 1938 and serves as a standard for general information about a wide range of assessment instruments.

We now turn to the case conceptualization process in clinical neuropsychology, a process that incorporates assessment findings with additional forms of information to assist the clinician's understanding of the patient's level of function.

FOUR

Case Formulation in Clinical Neuropsychology

The previous discussion of the historical background in clinical neuro-psychology is essential to our understanding of contemporary case formulation of the individual patient. This is because modern methods of "knowing" an individual patient—how he or she thinks, feels, and behaves—directly reflect the epistemological assumptions that have pervaded the field of clinical psychology and neuropsychology for at least a century. Specifically, two epistemological trends have largely evolved over the twentieth century and continue to underlie clinical neuropsychological case formulation today. The first trend, which incorporates and integrates *idiographic knowledge*, emphasizes how the individual is unique and distinct from the lives of others (Allport, 1961), even if it may be to the neglect of drawing inferences regarding how the individual's level of functioning compares with larger groups of individuals of similar backgrounds. The idiographic emphasis underlies the clinical neuropsychologist's common practice of beginning an evaluation with a relatively in-depth clinical interview, one that affords an opportunity to get to know the individual and generate hypotheses about how the patient's limitations (and strengths) may be distinct from others. A wealth of rich and meaningful data is collected during this interview process, and upon completion of the clinical interview the clinician is likely to have a sense of how and why the patient is struggling, as well as intuit how things might play out on formal testing.

The second epistemological trend, which emphasizes *nomothetic knowledge*, focuses on aspects of the human experience that are "lawful" or universal regardless of the individual patient under study. In certain specialized areas of medical practice such as neurology, the nomothetic assumption is that central nervous system dysfunction contributes to stereotypic pathological behavior patterns that directly follow the laws of physics for all persons. For instance, a stroke to certain brain regions typically results in predictable patterns of motor weakness, visual disturbance, or speech abnormality across all patient groups, regardless of age, gender, or cultural background. In clinical neuropsychology, the nomothetic assumption is that performances on cognitive measures should approximate a certain degree of normal variability among healthy individuals, and significant deviations from normal distributions of performance suggest impairment or cognitive dysfunction. Characterization of meaningful performance deviations is facilitated by comparing an individual's cognitive performances with large normative groups of similar background (e.g., according to age, education, gender). Interpretation of resultant standardized scores allows the clinician to understand varying levels of ability in various domains of cognitive functioning. Identification of the most fitting normative data (i.e., data that is are most consistent with the individual patient's background) represents an important component of respecting individuality and complementing it with what is expected relative to persons of similar demographic and cultural background (Nelson & Pontón, 2007; Strauss, Sherman, & Spreen, 2006).

Integration of individual-specific data (obtained through behavioral observations, the clinical interview, record review, collateral information from a significant other) and empirical norm-referenced data (obtained through formal testing) ultimately forms the foundation of case formulation in clinical neuropsychology. Attention to both quantitative and qualitative aspects of test data should also be given. As Boake (2008, p. 237) suggests: "competent neuropsychological evaluation requires that the clinician interpret test results both quantitatively, in terms of normative comparisons, and qualitatively, in terms of score profiles and error patterns." Convergent data obtained from these various areas of the patient's functioning are conceptualized and summarized through a formal report that provides feedback to the referral source and informs future treatment options that will ultimately be of benefit to the patient's future treatment and care (discussed further in chapter 6).

Clinical Neuropsychological Assessment as a Unique Evaluation Process

In clinical settings, the majority of referrals for neuropsychological evaluation come from physicians (such as a family or primary care physician) or from medical specialists (such as a neurologist, psychiatrist, or physiatrist) (Sweet, Nelson, & Moberg, 2006; Sweet et al., 2011). Implicit to the referral is an understanding that neuropsychologists have attained specialized training in the evaluation of cognitive function that physicians and other health care providers have not. For example, in geriatric settings, physicians are typically capable of recognizing moderate to severe dementias on the basis of performances on brief cognitive screening measures (e.g., Mini Mental State Examination), but tend to show more variable rates of detection in milder cases of dementia (van Hout et al., 2000; Olafsdottir, Skoog, & Marcussion, 2000). Similar data suggest that physical and occupational therapists' rates of detecting cognitive impairment are quite variable (Ruchinskas, 2002). Neuropsychologists are trained to detect not only severe forms of cognitive deficit, but also subtle deficits that may go undetected by the individual patient, family, or physicians and other health care providers (Lezak, 2003).

Neuropsychological evaluations not only document the level of cognitive impairment (if any), but may identify whether complaints of cognitive dysfunction are in fact corroborated by objective findings. Common applications of neuropsychological evaluation include providing a baseline level of cognitive status when longitudinal follow-up evaluation may be anticipated; assessing cognitive strengths or deficits that may be relevant to abilities in academic or occupational settings; assisting with differential diagnosis; and identifying strengths and weaknesses relevant to levels of functioning relevant to future rehabilitation and in terms of functional needs (Mitrushina et al., 2005). Neuropsychologists may also provide opinions regarding prognostic factors, how impairment might impact an individual's daily functioning, and offer appropriate treatment recommendations as needed. For instance, there is evidence that neuropsychological data have predictive value with regard to hospital lengths of stay (Galski et al., 1993), ability to maintain independent living (Lysack et al., 2003), or operate a motor vehicle (Reger et al., 2004). It is encouraging to note that neuropsychological impressions based upon objective test results have been found to be as valid as medical assessment of various conditions (Meyer et al., 2001).

The present chapter discusses case formulation by focusing on issues relevant to (1) assessment of response validity and effort, (2) assessment of cognitive functioning, (3) assessment of personality and emotional functioning, and (4) population-based case formulation.

Assessment of Response Validity and Effort

Neuropsychological test data must first be determined to be reliable before the data can be interpreted as reflecting a valid or accurate reflection of an individual's level of cognitive ability. To the extent that the patient is unwilling or unable to perform at potential during testing, the clinician's confidence in drawing conclusions relevant to cognitive status is attenuated. Performing at one's utmost potential during the testing process is essential to the inherent reliability and validity of neuropsychological test data. Just as sufficient effort during testing promotes performances on objective measures of cognitive ability, insufficient effort is known to diminish performances. As one illustration of the negative effect that insufficient effort may have on neuropsychological performances on ability measures, consider the findings of Green et al. (2001), who examined neuropsychological test performances among 904 individuals undergoing neuropsychological evaluation in various secondary gain contexts (e.g., personal injury litigation, worker's compensation, disability claim). The authors derived an overall test battery mean (OTBM) of cognitive ability based upon performances on several neuropsychological measures among participants. Dramatically, effort was found to correlate strongly with OTBM (. 73), and accounted for 4.5 times more variance in OTBM than moderate-severe traumatic brain injury itself!

The latter findings also illustrate that issues of insufficient effort, dissimulation of cognitive symptoms, and malingering are especially concerning in *forensic* settings. In routine *clinical* settings, a neuropsychologist is requested (usually by a physician or other fellow treating provider) to provide an evaluation of an individual's cognitive and psychological functioning related to clinical care and to inform appropriate treatment planning. In clinical settings, the neuropsychologist is working as a *treating provider* on behalf of the patient. In contrast, in a forensic setting, the neuropsychologist serves as an *expert* to render an opinion about the likelihood that an historical injury directly accounts for a litigant's or claimant's ongoing cognitive or psychological difficulties. Common forensic settings include personal injury litigation wherein a neuropsychologist is retained by an attorney, workers' compensation evaluations in which a neuropsychologist is consulted by an individual's employer to inform employability, or independent medical examinations in which a neuropsychologist is consulted by a disability insurance company to inform level of disability. In light of the strong external incentive that exists in forensic settings to appear more impaired than one actually is, secondary gain is especially prevalent in forensic settings. It is therefore not surprising that base rates of invalid self-presentation and malingering are estimated to be as high as 40% (Mittenberg et al., 2001b).

In light of findings like those of Mittenberg et al., 2001b), it is also not surprising that neuropsychologists are increasingly aware of the importance of first considering whether test data represent a reliable and accurate reflection of the patient's true level of cognitive ability before identifying the nature of "impaired" versus "intact" performances, particularly within forensic settings. Indeed, regardless of referral context (clinical or forensic), the issue of response validity assessment has been identified as an important practice guideline according to the American Academy of Clinical Neuropsychology: "The assessment of effort and motivation is important in any clinical setting, as a patient's effort may be compromised even in the absence of any potential or active litigation, compensation, or financial incentives" (; Heilbronner, 2007; p. 221).

Unfortunately, a literature review from the late 1970s to the early 1990s suggests that clinical neuropsychologists are largely ineffective in detecting insufficient effort on the basis of clinical intuition alone (Heaton et al., 1978; Schacter, 1986a, b; Faust, Hart, & Guilmette, 1988; Faust, Hart, Guilmette, & Arkes, 1988). In a classic study on this topic, Heaton et al. (1978) presented the neuropsychological profiles of 16 head-injured patients and 16 simulators (i.e., individuals instructed to perform suboptimally) to 10 clinical neuropsychologists for interpretation. The neuropsychologists were blinded to the conditions of interest, and were asked to identify those with genuine impairments and those who were known to be malingering. The neuropsychologists' identification of malingerers approximated chance-level performance, with only 50 to 68% of malingerers accurately identified. Additionally, the neuropsychologists were asked to rate the level of confidence that they had successfully identified those who were malingering, with results suggesting a weak correlation between level of confidence and classification accuracy. The findings of Schacter (1986a, b) and Faust et al. (1988a, b) were quite similar to the findings of Heaton et al. and revealed the humbling message that clinical intuition alone is insufficient in identifying patients who present themselves in a less than forthright manner.

In response to findings like these, an explosion of forensic neuropsychology literature has emerged since the early 1990s (Sweet, Moberg, & Suchy, 2000) and continues to address the topic of response validity assessment and malingering. Many of the studies that comprise this literature pertain to the development of specific measures that simultaneously demonstrate sensitivity to insufficient effort, as well as specificity with respect to genuine neurologic disorder and psychiatric illness.

Cognitive response validity measures in clinical neuropsychology may be classified according to two general categories: (1) Symptom Validity Tests (SVTs) developed for the sole purpose of identifying insufficient effort, and (2) Symptom Validity Indices (SVIs) that represent "embedded" effort indices that are retrospectively derived from standard measures of ability. Table 3.3 (see previous chapter) presents examples of just a few of the SVTs and SVIs that clinicians have at their disposal to assess response validity during neuropsychological evaluations. Thorough review of these measures and strategies of response validity assessment is beyond the scope of the current chapter, and the reader is encouraged to refer to the multitude of excellent references that provide a comprehensive discussion of forensic issues, including response validity and malingering in clinical neuropsychology (e.g., Boone, 2007; Morgan & Sweet, 2008; Strauss, Sherman, & Spreeen, 2006; Sweet, 1999).

Briefly, SVTs represent tasks whose sole basis for development is to detect whether an individual patient has put forth sufficient effort on testing. There are many SVTs to choose from, with two general classes that the clinician may rely upon: (1) non-forced-choice effort measures, and (2) forced-choice effort measures. The former class of SVT has existed for a greater number of years than the latter, with researchers such as Andre Rey being among the first to formulate measures that may assist in the response validity assessment process (e.g., the Rey-15 Item Test; the Rey Dot Counting Test). Forced-choice measures were born out of the pioneering work of Pankratz (1975), who applied forced-choice methodology to evaluate deafness among "hysterical" and malingering patients. According to this methodology, performance on a given two-alternative forced-choice task should approximate 50% correct on the basis of random responding alone. Thus, a performance that is statistically and significantly below chance in the forced-choice paradigm suggests that the patient was aware of the correct responses and opted to endorse the incorrect responses with some level of intentionality (see Millis, 2004 for a review of forced-choice methodology and application of the binomial probability theory). In recognition of the fact that statistically significantly less-than-chance performance is a relatively rare phenomenon, optimal cut-scores have been identified on forced-choice measures that are above the chance level, but nevertheless optimal in the detection of insufficient effort (see Boone, 2007; Strauss, Sherman, Spreen, 2006).

SVIs have been derived across the cognitive domains of orientation/attention, language, motor, executive, and learning/memory functioning (see Table 3.3 for examples). Most SVIs rely on a floor effect strategy in the identification of insufficient effort. That is, performances that are identified to be well beneath what is typically observed even among the most severely impaired patients (e.g., those with dementia) are interpreted as implicating insufficient effort. In general, SVIs retain excellent specificity relative to most clinical conditions (i.e., relatively strong true negative rates for insufficient effort), but often show limited sensitivity (i.e., relatively limited true positive rates for identification of insufficient effort). Most clinicians agree that this arrangement (i.e., strong specificity at the expense of weak sensitivity) is "safer" than the alternative of maximizing sensitivity at the expense of specificity given the relatively high cost that may follow in the wake of incorrectly identifying a given patient as malingering. Caution should be exercised, however, for certain clinical groups (e.g., patients with mental retardation) in which a higher rate of false positive identifications has been demonstrated (see Boone, 2007).

When incorporated with relevant background information, SVTs and SVIs may be implemented to support a diagnosis of factitious disorder or malingering, conditions that according to DSM-IV-TR require evidence that symptoms have been *intentionally* feigned or exaggerated. In the case of factitious disorder, symptoms are intentionally feigned for primary gain purposes (i.e., to maintain a sick role). In the case of malingering, symptoms are intentionally feigned for secondary gain purposes (e.g., to obtain financial remuneration or avoid military service). DSM-IV-TR suggests that malingering should be considered in medico-legal contexts, when individuals present with features consistent with antisocial personality disorder, for example. However, this scheme has been noted to have limited use in neuropsychology, and an alternative diagnostic scheme that is frequently relied upon are the guidelines for malingered neurocognitive dysfunction (MND) provided by Slick et al. (1999). According to this scheme, among claimants who are known to be involved in litigation or evaluated in other secondary gain contexts, varying levels of performance support possible MND, probable MND, and definitive MND at varying levels of performance on SVTs and/or SVIs. As mentioned, statistically significantly less-than-chance performance on a forced-choice measure suggests at least some degree of intentional identification of incorrect responses, and Slick et al. (1999) have suggested that less-than-chance performance on a forced-choice measure is the closest to an "evidentiary gold standard of malingering" that is available. However, it is worth noting that a healthy debate continues to play out on this issue, with some suggesting that effort measures are not capable of measuring intention (even in the case of less-than-chance performance on a forced-choice measure), and others suggesting that intention may be inferred from such a pattern of performance. The reader should be aware that the construct of "malingering" is an evolving one, and in light of recent debates it is hoped that criteria will undergo modification in DSM-V (Berry & Nelson, 2010).

For present purposes, the fundamental message is that the validity of neuropsychological test results cannot be determined until results have first been identified as being reliable. Just as an MMPI-2 profile should not be interpreted as reflecting an accurate reflection of a patient's psychological/emotional state until it has first been determined that the profile is valid (according to validity scales), so the neuropsychological profile should not be interpreted as accurate until it has first been determined that the patient put forth sufficient effort during the course of testing. Only then is the clinician able to draw conclusions pertinent to level of functioning (impaired versus intact) according to the various domains of cognitive functioning, to which we now turn.

Assessment of Cognitive Functioning

TEST SELECTION, PRE-MORBID BACKGROUND, AND DEMOGRAPHIC CONSIDERATIONS

There are hundreds of measures that the neuropsychologist may consider in assessing a given patient's cognitive strengths and weaknesses, and dozens of new measures appear each year (Lezak, 2003). Standardized measures are usually preferable to other less well-developed measures to minimize error variance that may surround individual performances (Miller & Rohling, 2001). Clinicians should be familiar with the psychometric properties that underlie the measures that they administer and refrain from administering tests with which they have little familiarity (American Psychological Association, 2002).

It should also be noted that "standard" measures typically support a greater level of confidence regarding a patient's abilities relative to "experimental" measures. Mitrushina et al. (2005) suggest that at a minimum, three of four criteria should be met before a measure should be understood as being in standard use:

- First, the test should be widely accessible to the professional community and have adequate normative data to support generation of standardized scores.

- Second, the test stimulus and materials should be standardized, and should include a manual that describes how measures are to be administered. Reliability and validity data should also be available to verify that the measure is psychometrically sound.

- Third, research with use of the test should be peer-reviewed and published in recognized professional journals. In this way, the measure has demonstrated a level of acceptance by the professional community at large.

- Finally, the test should have been reviewed in the *Mental Measurements Yearbook* or in neuropsychological texts by authors who are not directly affiliated with the measure (Mitrushina et al., 2005).

As discussed in chapter 3, neuropsychologists continue to implement a flexible battery approach to test administration (Sweet et al., 2011), which entails administration of several core measures complemented by other measures depending upon an individual's specific presenting difficulties. Regardless of the approach employed, test selection is likely to depend upon the specific referral question or diagnostic purposes. For example, for a patient referred for neuropsychological evaluation of possible dementia, the clinician is likely to administer a number of learning/memory tasks as well as select measures from other cognitive domains to allow for formal diagnosis of dementia according to DSM-IV-TR (which requires evidence of impairment in memory function as well as at least one other cognitive domain).

Most clinicians recognize the importance of considering the patient's *pre-morbid background* when considering test selection and when conceptualizing individual neuropsychological profiles. Consideration of such factors as early developmental neurologically relevant events (e.g., complicated birth, childhood head injury), conditions that impact academic achievement (e.g., childhood learning disability, attention-deficit), and level of academic attainment (e.g., high school versus college-educated) can significantly impact the clinician's understanding of a patient's cognitive limitations. Evidence of pre-morbid limitations disclosed during the clinical interview might prompt administration of measures that might not have been otherwise administered. For example, if a patient reports a longstanding difficulty in mathematical ability, it would likely be prudent to administer a basic measure of mathematical achievement (e.g., WRAT-IV, Written Arithmetic) before administering or interpreting measures of cognitive function that rely upon over-learned arithmetic ability (e.g., Paced Auditory Serial Addition Test).

Various strategies have also been developed to estimate levels of pre-morbid intellectual functioning. Such estimates may assist the clinician to conceptualize whether a patient's current level of cognitive function represents a significant decline from pre-morbid function in the wake of brain injury or other issue relevant to cognitive function. Some of these strategies simply rely upon the individual patient's demographic background information. For example, estimates of pre-morbid full, verbal, and performance IQ abilities may be generated according to an individual's age, gender, race, level of education, occupation, and living environment (e.g., Barona, Reynolds, & Chastain, 1984). Other strategies rely upon the patient's ability to identify written words to estimate pre-morbid intelligence (e.g., Wechsler Test of Adult Reading or WTAR, Psychological Corporation, 2001), with the conceptual understanding that the capacity to identify written words is one that is often resistant to brain injury. Still other strategies incorporate demographic background and select intellectual performances to estimate pre-morbid level of intelligence (e.g., Oklahoma Pre-morbid Intelligence Estimate or OPIE-3; Schoenberg et al., 2002; 2003). Regardless of the approach, consideration of where the patient has been and what the patient has achieved prior to the neuropsychological evaluation is an important consideration in most cases to inform the likelihood that certain impaired performances may or may not reflect pre-morbid limitations as opposed to, say, a recent traumatic brain injury or other brain-related event. It should be noted that these pre-morbid estimates do have limitations, which might in part account for their variable use in routine clinical practice (Smith-Seemiller et al., 1997).

In interpreting cognitive performances, neuropsychologists also recognize that certain *demographic* variables often impact performances on objective measures, and this warrants adjustment of raw score performances to standardized performances derived from large normative groups. Normative data are typically stratified by age, gender, level of educational attainment, and at times ethnicity (refer to Mitrushina et al., 2005; Strauss, Sherman, & Spreen, 2006). Age is among the most well researched demographic variables known to impact neuropsychological performances, with at least some degree of decline to be expected on the basis of normal aging alone (Haaland, Price, & Larue, 2003). Level of education often shows a strong relationship with performances across the domains of cognitive function, which warrants stratification on the basis of educational attainment (Heatonet al., 2004).

THEORETICAL ASSUMPTIONS RELEVANT TO CASE CONCEPTUALIZATION

The basic domains of cognitive functioning routinely assessed in contemporary neuropsychology are born out of a rich and fascinating history of cognitive and intellectual theory (see McGrew, 1997). Cognitive domains typically include overall intellectual functioning, level of orientation, attention/concentration, speech/language, visual-spatial functioning, executive functioning, sensorimotor functioning, and learning/memory. Table 3.3, in the previous chapter, depicts some of the most frequently administered measures that neuropsychologists rely upon. We refer the reader to other more comprehensive texts for a complete review of the many measures that facilitate assessment of these various cognitive domains (see Strauss, Sherman, & Spreen, 2006; Lezak et al., 2004; Mitrushina et al., 2005).

One explanation for the many neuropsychological measures available to the clinician relates to the theoretical heterogeneity that underlies the various cognitive domains; within each cognitive domain of interest there exist multiple distinct subdomains of function. Thus, within the domain of attention/concentration there exist such constructs as simple versus complex attention, sustained versus divided attention, vigilance, and reaction time. Evaluation of speech and language processing typically follows the theoretical elements that characterize the classic aphasias. Hence, many neuropsychological evaluations include measures of verbal expression (fluency), receptive language (comprehension), repetition, and naming ability. The realm of executive functioning is arguably the most diverse of cognitive domains, which may speak to the complexity of frontal systems networks that facilitate complex planning and behaviors. Executive measures include tasks relevant to abstraction, concept formation, the ability to benefit from external feedback, planning and organization, spontaneity, response inhibition, and other higher order conceptual processes. The construct of learning and memory may be further classified according to auditory versus visual memory components, with differential performances in these areas potentially suggesting lateralized brain dysfunction. Neuropsychologists recognize that no single measure is capable of fully representing an individual's level of ability in a given domain, and interpretation of multiple performances within a domain allows for a more robust understanding of the complexity of function within that area.

Also, these theoretical cognitive domains are not necessarily mutually exclusive. For example, verbal fluency tasks (semantic and phonemic) entail the rapid generation of words from a given category in a designated period of time. Verbal fluency may be regarded as a measure of language function, but might also be construed as an executive task in the sense that it entails spontaneous and efficient production of information while simultaneously activating response inhibition (e.g., the ability to refrain from repeating oneself; avoidance of words outside of the class requested). Many clinicians rely upon the Wechsler Adult Intelligence Scale–Fourth Edition (WAIS-IV) and other broadband measures to evaluate not only overall level of intellectual ability, but to describe performances relevant to various other domains of cognitive function. The various WAIS-III subtests include diverse cognitive components that are typically described not only in the realm of intellectual functioning, but with respect to underlying cognitive factors of verbal comprehension (vocabulary, similarities, information), perceptual organization (picture completion, block design, matrix reasoning), working memory (digit span, letter-numbers sequencing, arithmetic), and processing speed (digit-symbol coding, symbol search). In the process of reporting neuropsychological test findings, a clinician may refer to a given test performance within more than one cognitive domain.

The overlapping nature of cognitive constructs is also relevant to the observation that certain cognitive domains are fundamental to others, and impairment in one domain may be the direct result of impairment in another. For example, evidence of intact arousal and attention is necessary before the clinician can reliably evaluate other domains of cognitive function. A patient who is clearly delirious and unable to sustain attention in conversation for even brief periods of time is likely to demonstrate impairment on nearly every measure administered (attention, learning/memory, language, etc.). In this scenario, it is likely prudent for the clinician to refrain from interpreting impairments in learning/memory as memory impairment per se, given that attention is the more fundamental issue that underlies the impairment. Similarly, fundamental sensory processes, regardless of modality, need to be intact before higher levels of cognitive functioning within the same modality can be reliably evaluated. It would be erroneous to interpret verbal learning/memory performances in a deaf patient, visual memory performances in a blind patient, or motor performances in a patient with restricted use of the hands.

Finally, domains outside of the cognitive realm may impact cognitive function and are therefore also routinely evaluated. Effort/motivation, though not a cognitive domain per se, is nevertheless essential to a patient's ability to demonstrate reliable performances on neuropsychological measures of ability, and is therefore frequently evaluated through *symptom validity testing*. Psychological and emotional symptoms such as depression or anxiety may contribute not only to a subjective experience of cognitive limitation, but also to impaired performances on objective measures (e.g., cognitive efficiency, attention, learning/memory). It is therefore not surprising that measures of personality and emotional functioning, such as the Minnesota Multiphasic Personality Inventory–2nd Edition (MMPI-2; Butcher et al., 1989), are administered nearly as frequently as measures of neuropsychological function (Camara, Nathan, & Puente, 2000; Rabin, Barr, & Burton, 2005).

Assessment of Personality and Emotional Functioning

Holistic neuropsychological evaluation includes a thorough assessment of cognitive status, as well as psychological and emotional functioning. In clinical neuropsychology, an understanding of the patient's personality and emotional status is important not only to explore whether symptoms may be significant enough to support a formal psychological diagnosis, but also to detect whether psychological symptoms may be sufficiently severe to account for objective cognitive impairment. As noted previously, physicians and other health care providers have shown variable rates of detecting subtle cognitive limitations among their patients (van Hout et al., 2000; Olafsdottir et al., 2000); primary care providers have also shown variable rates of detecting mood disorders among their patients (Klinkman, 1997; Garrard, Rolnick, & Nitz, 1998). This further emphasizes the importance of making appropriate referrals for neuropsychological evaluation when cognitive and emotional symptoms are expressed simultaneously. In particular, neuropsychologists' concurrent interpretation of cognitive and emotional functioning may clarify the full constellation of symptoms (cognitive, behavioral, and psychological) that may be associated with a host of neurologic conditions (e.g., Huntington's disease, Parkinson's disease, multiple sclerosis).

As an illustration of the importance of concurrent evaluation of psychological and cognitive functioning in geriatric groups, some literature suggests that patients with co-morbid cognitive and psychological symptoms demonstrate greater levels of disability relative to patients with either symptom set alone. In a geriatric sample, Forsell and Winblad (1998) found that while dementia itself increases disability, level of disability was even greater among dementia groups who were also depressed. Espiritu et al. (2001) reported similar findings in their sample of 141 geriatric outpatients referred for evaluation of memory difficulty. Seventy percent of the group met criteria for probable Alzheimer's dementia, and more than 60% of the sample showed indication of functional impairment. A multiple regression analysis suggested that cognition (MMSE) accounted for 18% total variance as a predictor of functional status, and emotional symptoms (Geriatric Depression Scale) accounted for 23% total variance in the prediction of functional status. Findings suggested that depression was related to functional status beyond what could be accounted for by cognitive impairment alone.

It is also important to recognize that while psychological symptoms may contribute to objective cognitive performances for some individuals, the patient's subjective experience of cognitive limitation does not necessarily translate to objective cognitive impairment on formal neuropsychological testing. For instance, some degree of diminished cognitive efficiency or memory functioning is expected on the basis of aging alone, and for some individuals, complaints of diminished cognitive functioning may simply represent a normal aging process. In others, cognitive complaints represent a manifestation of significant psychiatric symptoms. DSM-IV-TR states that subjective experience of diminished attention/concentration is a supportive criterion for formal diagnosis of major depressive disorder, even if there is not objective evidence of attentional impairment on formal testing. Numerous studies have demonstrated a relatively weak relationship between self-reported cognitive limitations and objective cognitive test findings. Otto et al. (1994) examined the effects of depressive symptoms on memory functioning and found that self-reported cognitive problems were significantly related to depression severity without consistent indication of objective cognitive impairment on formal testing. Similarly, Derouesne et al. (1999) studied memory complaints in young and elderly healthy groups and found that both groups showed little relationship between memory complaints and objective memory performance. Both groups showed strong relationships between memory complaints and affective state (primarily anxiety), even though neither group was clinically depressed or anxious.

There are many well-validated measures of personality and emotional functioning to consider, and clinical neuropsychologists typically administer the same measures that general clinical psychologists rely upon. The MMPI-2 (Butcher et al., 1989) continues to be the most widely administered personality inventory among clinical neuropsychologists (Rabin et al., 2005), though other personality inventories such as the Personality Assessment Inventory (PAI; Morey, 1991) are also in frequent use. The reader is probably aware that the benefit of the latter two inventories is their inclusion of validity scales that assist the clinician in identifying random responding, under-endorsement and over-endorsement of psychological symptoms, as well as a number of clinical scales and subscales that effectively discriminate diagnostic groups and inform treatment recommendations. Briefer measures of emotional functioning include face valid self-report measures such as the Beck Depression Inventory – 2nd Edition (BDI-II, Beck, Steer, & Brown, 1996) or for elder groups the Geriatric Depression Scale (GDS, Brink et al., 1982). We refer the reader to other references relevant to interpretation of personality inventories and self-report measures for a complete review of these instruments and interpretation strategies (Strauss, Sherman, & Spreen, 2006; Lezak et al., 2004.

Population-Based Case Formulation and Base Rates

After raw score performances have been obtained within each of the cognitive domains of interest, they are typically transformed to standardized scores (e.g., T-score, z-score) based upon key demographic stratifying variables (e.g., age, education). These standardized scores then provide the basis for the clinician's description of various levels of performance (e.g., impaired, average, superior). Impairment is typically identified with a certain level of statistical deviation from mean performance in a normative sample. Heaton et al. (2004), for example, offer descriptors of varying levels of impairment beginning at T-scores of 40 or less, or one standard deviation below mean level of performance in the normative sample. Other schemes, such as those described by Lezak et al. (2004), Mitrushina et al. (2005), and Strauss, Sherman, and Spreen (2006), identify impairment at the 9th percentile or less, or approximately 1.3 standard deviations below the normative mean. Thus, impairment is usually identified with performance that ranges from 1.3 to 1.0 standard deviations below normative mean performance.

However, clinicians show variability in how they describe and conceive of standardized score performances, including what constitutes an objectively impaired performance. Guilmette et al. (2008) surveyed a sample of 110 board-certified clinical neuropsychologists to determine use of qualitative performance descriptors in forensic and non-forensic contexts across a range of performances. Participants were asked to assign descriptors to 12 different standard scores (SS) ranging from 50 to 130. Overall, greater consistency was observed in describing higher SS than lower SS. For example, 61.5% of the sample used the same qualitative descriptor when SS was greater than 80, while only one third of the sample used the same descriptive label for SS ranging from 50 to 75.

It is also important for neuropsychologists to recognize the great amount of intraindividual variability that exists in healthy samples on neuropsychological measures (Schretlen et al., 2003), and that a meaningful proportion of healthy samples demonstrate isolated impaired performances that cannot be clearly attributed to underlying brain dysfunction (Palmer et al., 1998; Schretlen et al., 2008). Using a broad battery of measures, Palmer et al. (1998) examined base rates of impaired neuropsychological performances in a sample of healthy older adults. Across measures, participants showed some proportion of borderline to impaired range performance (1.3 and 2.0 standard deviations below the age-group mean, respectively). Nearly three quarters of participants demonstrated borderline performance on at least one measure, and 20% of participants demonstrated two scores that were within an impaired range on separate tests.

In a study of neuropsychological performances in a sample of healthy community participants, Schretlen et al. (2008) found that approximately 75% showed two or more performances that were at or below a T-score of 40 when administered 25 measures, while approximately 36% of participants showed two or more performances below this same level when administered 10 cognitive measures. The latter findings suggest that test length may impact rates of deficient performance.

Findings like those reported by Palmer et al. (1998) and Schretlen et al. (2008) highlight the wide variability in performance that exists in healthy individuals in terms of neuropsychological performance. The neuro-psychologist should exercise caution in attempting to correlate an isolated deviant performance with underlying neurologic disturbance. Neuropsychologists also recognize that base rates of a given condition in a given clinical condition may vary by evaluation context. Awareness of measurement sensitivities, specificities, and positive and negative predictive validities in specific evaluation contexts should be considered when interpreting performances and drawing diagnostic conclusions. We refer the reader to other available references for a more detailed review of these issues (McCaffrey et al., 2003; Smith, Ivnik, & Lucas, 2008).

Conclusion

Case conceptualization in clinical neuropsychological evaluation entails assessment of cognitive, behavioral, and emotional functioning according to performances on well validated standardized measures that are considered within the individual patient's unique demographic and cultural background. Integration of information that is unique to the patient with norm-referenced data allows the examiner to attain a uniform and comprehensive understanding of the patient and his or her areas of functional strength and weakness. These various forms of information are described in detail through the medium of neuropsychological report writing, the topic to which we now turn.

PART III

Functional Competency— Report Writing

FIVE

The Neuropsychological Evaluation Report

Now that we have explored some of the general guidelines that inform case conceptualization and formulation in the neuropsychological evaluation (chapter 4), we are able to discuss in detail how these topics may be effectively applied in clinical practice, specifically through the medium of neuropsychological report writing. The current chapter provides a relatively brief overview of elements included in clinical neuropsychological report writing. We recommend a variety of additional resources that explore the art of report writing and related topics for further reference (Axelrod, 2000; Lezak et al., 2004; Ownby, 1997; Sattler, 1992; Strauss, Sherman, & Spreen, 2006).

Report Writing

There is not one single strategy or method of report writing that is necessarily superior to another; there is no "cookbook approach" (Vanderploeg, 2000). Variations in report format, report length, grammatical preference, and subtle (and sometimes rather interesting) idiosyncrasies in report writing abound. Boake (2008, p. 237) suggests that "neuropsychological evaluation varies according to the purpose, the needs of the referral source, the clinician's approach, and the time available." It follows that information included in a formal neuropsychological evaluation report will also vary. For example, the clinical context may determine the length, format, and content of the report. Outpatient reports may include greater elaboration upon self-reported history than inpatient reports, the latter of which may simply refer the reader to medical records for a complete review of the patient's background and circumstances leading up to a hospitalization and referral for evaluation. Forensic reports are more likely to include extended review of external records verifying a given brain-related event (e.g., traumatic brain injury) purported to contribute to the claimant's cognitive limitations than clinical reports, which are more likely to provide a relatively brief summary of records that may be relevant to the patient's current limitations. The physician who is familiar with a given patient may even simply request that the neuropsychologist provide a brief summary of cognitive test findings through a brief progress note rather than generate a formal neuropsychological report.

As an illustration of the diversity that exists among neuropsychologists in their routine report writing, consider the findings of Donders (2001a, b), who conducted a survey of Division 40 members of the American Psychological Association (APA) on this topic. Survey data from 414 neuropsychologists (approximately 11% of APA Division 40 membership at that time) suggested that certain aspects of report writing are strikingly uniform across practice settings. The great majority of respondents indicated that they include such variables as the patient's age, gender, handedness, level of education, previous neurological history, prior substance abuse, current medications, and employment history always or routinely in their neuropsychological reports. Greater than 94% of the sample indicated that they routinely or always include information about the referral source, the reason for evaluation, a description of clinical presentation, a summary of measures administered, and a description of test performances in descriptive terms. Nearly 78% of neuropsychologists indicated that they always separate unique background information into distinct sections (e.g., patient history, observations, test results), and an additional 21% indicated that they routinely do so.

However, less uniformity was observed on a variety of other variables (Donders, 2001a, b). Findings suggested marked variability of reporting which normative data or normative procedures were used to analyze test data, with board-certified respondents more than twice as likely to exclude this information as respondents without board certification. Approximately 18% of the sample indicated that they never included information pertaining to history of previous litigation or other financial compensation-seeking in their reports, while more than 12% of the sample indicated that they always did. Not surprisingly, patient age was found to moderate this variable, with significantly fewer pediatric reports exploring the issue of prior compensation-seeking (given that children are less likely to have a history of prior secondary gain issues relative to adults). In short, these relatively recent survey data suggest that while there is relative uniformity among neuropsychologists regarding many aspects of report writing, other areas may vary depending upon the background of the individual clinician and patient.

EFFECTIVE REPORT WRITING STRATEGIES

Regardless of the precise content and stylistic strategy employed in report writing, neuropsychological reports that express ideas clearly are the most effective and helpful to the reader. Careful attention should be given to language and wording, and use of psychological jargon should be avoided whenever possible (Strauss, Sherman, & Spreen, 2006). When technical language is used in reports, the clinician should consider elaborating to maximize the likelihood that the reader (who could very well be the patient under discussion) will understand the message conveyed. For example, when describing performance on a measure of phonemic fluency, the clinician should consider an additional descriptor that summarizes the task, such as "a measure that entails efficient generation of words beginning with a given letter." Rather than simply referring to performance on a measure of verbal memory, it is helpful to clarify that this entails "recall of story details," and so on. In so doing, the neuropsychologist effectively bridges information that is a given to certain readers with what is new to others (Ownby, 1997).

Further, reports that follow a logical sequence of thought are usually the most compelling to the reader (Axelrod, 2000; Ownby, 1990, 1997). Thus, it is logical that most neuropsychological reports begin with a brief statement as to why the neuropsychological evaluation was requested before a detailed description of self-report cognitive limitations and objective test findings is provided. It is logical that a complete summarization of objective test results is provided according to the various domains of cognitive function before test results are interpreted and applied within the diagnostic impressions section. It is only after an opinion has been made regarding diagnosis/prognosis that the clinician is able to complete the report by providing treatment recommendations or suggested modifications that bear upon the patient's everyday functioning.

It is also important to recognize that no report can be regarded as being completely objective in nature, which is why the referral source is seeking the expert's *opinion* about cognitive status based upon available information. Conceptualization of findings may vary related to the amount of information available and the clinician's level of training, knowledge base, understanding of the neuropsychology literature, and opinion regarding what differentiates normal and abnormal cognitive function. Recognition of one's own personal (that is, subjective) viewpoints and experiential limitations may serve to minimize bias or prejudice during the report writing process (Sattler, 1992).

Individual differences aside, most neuropsychological reports explore a number of fundamental areas that collectively support a well-rounded summary of the individual patient's background, current level of functioning, and implications for future care. Neuropsychological reports are likely to include most or all of the following elements:

(1) Brief statement describing the referral source and the rationale for evaluation

(2) Behavioral observations

(3) Background information obtained in the clinical interview

(4) Collateral information obtained from an individual familiar with the patient

(5) Review of relevant available records

(6) Test results across the domains of cognitive and personality/ emotional functioning

(7) Diagnostic impressions

(8) Treatment recommendations.

Emphasis in any one of these areas may vary depending upon:

• information that may or may not be available to the clinician (e.g., many versus few available outside records),

• time available prior to delivery of the report (e.g., hours in the case of last-minute inpatient consult versus weeks in the case of some independent medical evaluations),

• accuracy of self-report information (e.g., whether the patient is a relatively good or poor historian),

• the patient's tolerance for the testing process (e.g., according to age, level of function, degree of disability, level of cooperation),

• a host of potential co-morbid conditions that may warrant elaborate exploration (e.g., co-morbid chronic mental illness and neurodegenerative dementia),

• the setting in which the evaluation occurs (e.g., inpatient versus outpatient context),

- and the clinician's opinion with regard to the minimum amount of information that is needed to provide a fair documentation of the patient's level of function.

The systematic integration of these various content areas is ultimately what makes neuropsychological assessment distinct from (and more comprehensive than) neuropsychological testing (Vanderploeg, 2000).

The Referral Source and Rationale for Neuropsychological Evaluation

Prior to the time of the initial meeting for neuropsychological evaluation, it is usually beneficial for the examiner to have an understanding of the referral source (e.g., primary care provider, social worker, neurologist, psychiatrist), how and why the patient came to be referred for evaluation, and what specific questions the referral source or the patient may have with respect to cognitive/emotional/behavioral status and related functioning in everyday life. The spectrum of potential referral questions may range from quite specific on one end of the extreme (e.g., "does the patient's memory complaint seem consistent with Alzheimer's disease?") to rather general or even vague on the other (e.g., "please assess"). Often, the clinician is able to develop at least a cursory understanding of the referred patient's background information through record review that may be available within the patient's medical chart or records provided or retrieved from an outside institution.

At other times, information regarding the patient's background or even why the patient was referred for evaluation at all may not be available to the examiner. In this circumstance, it is usually helpful to contact the referral source to clarify and specify the question of interest. When this is not possible, the neuropsychologist might infer the reason for referral based upon available records or the patient's presenting complaints. The clinician might also identify issues relevant to cognitive and functional abilities that were not clearly evident to the referral source and may find it important to include these issues within the evaluation and formal report. In other words: "the neuropsychologist should answer not only the referral questions that were asked, but also those *that should have been asked*" (Vanderploeg, 2000, p. 7, emphasis added).

It should also be noted that the appropriateness of any referral is left to the discretion of the clinician. A patient with ongoing experience of florid hallucination associated with a lifelong paranoid schizophrenia referred for evaluation of possible ADHD would be an example of a poor referral question. The clinician may also identify factors from the patient's background (e.g., untreated sleep apnea, continued use of illicit substances) that might warrant greater management before the patient undergoes the neuropsychological evaluation. In general, the more that the clinician has learned about the individual patient prior to the neuropsychological evaluation proper, the more efficient the clinician will be in conducting the neuropsychological evaluation and preparing the neuropsychological evaluation report.

With these considerations in mind, most neuropsychological reports begin with a brief statement of the patient's background (e.g., name, age, gender) and the reason for referral. A concise statement about the patient and the referral is an efficient means of setting the stage for what follows in the other areas of the report, and for the informed reader initiates the hypothesis-generation process. For instance, suppose that a clinician introduces the report with the following statement about the patient's reason for referral: "Mr. Smith is a 60-year-old, nonfamilial left-handed, college-educated, African American widower referred for neuropsychological evaluation of a five-year history of progressive memory decline." In this one relatively concise statement, one is able to identify a number of factors that may potentially bear upon the patient's cognitive status. Progressive memory decline with onset in one's mid-50s raises the possibility of an early stage of Alzheimer's disease or other neurodegenerative process. Nonfamilial left-handedness raises the notion of possible brain insult early in neurodevelopment. Knowledge of the patient's college education provides a context regarding the possibility of cognitive reserve and its relationship to cognitive limitation with age. The patient's ethnic background could be relevant to literature that suggests a higher base rate of stroke among African Americans. That the patient is a widower raises the question of when his partner expired and whether the course of memory difficulty coincides with bereavement or a primary mood disorder. In short, a statement regarding the referral question and its rationale efficiently communicates the circumstances of the evaluation and provides a foundation for what follows in other sections of the report.

Behavioral Observations

Behavioral observations obtained during the clinical interview and testing session are often helpful in providing clues about what might be anticipated on formal testing and what limitations the patient may exhibit in everyday life. This section of the report may also serve as an introduction to factors that may have relevance to objective performances on formal measures. A clinician may include information obtained during brief mental examination within the behavioral observations section, and discuss how the patient's level of arousal, orientation, attention, motivation, or fatigue during testing may relate to the ecological utility of test findings (Axelrod, 2000). Behavioral observations provide the clinician with a first impression regarding issues relevant to self-care, ambulation and movement, quality of speech and language, mood and emotional state, and ability to follow through with requests during testing. Observational data regarding the patient's recognition of cognitive, emotional, or behavioral issues also provide essential information regarding insight into one's overall level of functioning. Frequently employed terms to describe behavior can be helpful in providing a skeleton on which to hang one's observations. For example, in discussion of the patient's overall level of arousal, the clinician may refer to terms such as "fully oriented and responsive" on one end of the spectrum, to "somnolent," "lethargic," "obtunded," or "comatose" at the other end of the spectrum. These are well-recognized terms that are likely to facilitate for the informed reader an understanding of what it was the clinician observed during the evaluation. However, these descriptors may not be helpful for individuals who are not accustomed to such terminology (such as the patient himself). Thus, it may be helpful to describe the patient according to technical terms, and then proceed to provide examples of what was observed to further express the unique nature of the individual patient's behavior. As one illustration, rather than simply stating that the patient's speech was significant for "paraphasic errors" in conversation, the clinician might consider stating that "the patient presented with intermittent paraphasic errors during the clinical interview and at one point referred to a pencil as a stencil."

PRESENTATION AND DEMEANOR

The behavioral observations section of the report often begins with a general statement regarding the patient's overall *presentation* and *demeanor*. Did the patient arrive on time? If not, what were the circumstances that contributed to his/her tardiness? Did the patient arrive unaccompanied or with a significant other? The clinician might comment as to whether the patient appears older or younger than the stated age. Observations of dress and grooming are often made; was the patient neatly or casually dressed and was dress appropriate to the situation? A statement regarding overall build (thin, average, slender, overweight, well nourished) may be provided. Description of overall grooming can provide initial clues regarding the patient's ability or interest in maintaining self-care (well groomed, neglected, or disheveled). Among individuals with difficulties abstaining from substance abuse, the clinician might be mindful of whether the smell of alcohol or other substance is present, and if so whether this may preclude formal testing.

GAIT AND MOVEMENT

Initial impressions regarding the quality of the patient's *gait* and *movement* provide preliminary information regarding possible brain involvement or other issues quite unrelated to brain dysfunction. Regarding the former, the patient may exhibit unilateral motor weakness as a result of a stroke that may provide hints regarding localized brain disturbance. Gait instability may represent a manifestation of Parkinson's disease or of a normal pressure hydrocephalus. Resting tremor of the hands may also reflect extrapyramidal brain involvement, while tremor with movement or action may correlate with cerebellar involvement. Atypical or involuntary movements may represent medication effect or a withdrawal symptom (as in the case of benzodiazepine withdrawal). Observations of movement may also inform issues unrelated to brain disturbance. Restricted movement associated with a recent back fusion or carpal tunnel surgery provides the reader with information that may limit the patient's ability to perform select tasks during formal testing. Motoric tendencies may also represent a manifestation of anxiety (fidgetiness), depression (overall slowing or delayed response latencies), or hypomania (hyperactivity). Stereotypic postures may be associated with an underlying psychotic process as in the case of catatonic schizophrenia.

SPEECH AND LANGUAGE

The quality of the patient's *speech* and *language* can be quite informative, and many clinicians summarize each dimension of language functioning used to categorize the aphasias (addressing receptive and expressive language elements). For example:

- How well does the patient comprehend what is discussed in conversation?
- What is the quality of articulation (clear, slurred, dysarthric)?
- Is speech prosodic or monotonic?
- Is rate of speech normal, slowed, pressured?
- Does the patient seem to be a good historian and provide a relatively accurate account of background information as corroborated by the collateral interview with a significant other or record review?

- Does the patient respond to interview questions openly and appropriately, or is he/she tangential and difficult to re-direct to topics of interest?
- Are perseverative tendencies present?
- Are word-finding difficulties for the specific names of significant others present?

Observations about speech and language may provide information regarding possible brain involvement or factors that are more likely associated with psychiatric disorder. Observations regarding fluency and comprehension during the clinical interview may provide convergent data in support of a formal receptive/expressive aphasia related to historical stroke or a language-based dementia (e.g., primary progressive aphasia or semantic dementia). Rapid rate of speech may relate to anxiety and slowed rate of speech may relate to depressive symptoms.

MOOD AND AFFECT

A description of *mood* and *affect* is very helpful, particularly when considered conjointly with results of formal measures of personality and emotional testing. Conventionally, mood pertains to the patient's subjective experience of emotional functioning and can be easily obtained by asking how the patient has been feeling recently (perhaps within the last few days or weeks). Affect pertains to the clinician's observation of the patient's emotional state. Mood may be described as euthymic (normal), depressed, anxious, irritable, angry, and so on. Affect may be restricted, constricted, tense, shallow, euphoric, or otherwise. Description of mood relative to affect allows for a statement of mood congruence versus incongruence and an understanding of the patient's insight into emotional functioning. For example, a patient who is frequently tearful during the clinical interview and describes herself as depressed would suggest mood congruence. Differently, the patient who is tearful but describes himself as feeling "just fine" or "happy" would suggest mood incongruence and perhaps diminished insight into emotional functioning.

RELATIONSHIP TO THE EXAMINER AND
APPROACH TO TASKS

The patient's *relationship to the examiner* and *approach to presented tasks* may bear relevance to objective performances during the testing session. Did the patient relate to the examiner in a respectful manner? Did the patient express interest and curiosity about what the tasks might be assessing? Alternatively, was the patient rude during testing or inappropriately flirtatious? Was the patient generally cooperative with the test administrator or reluctant to perform at potential? Based upon observation alone (i.e., independent of performances on effort measures), did the patient appear to put forth a concerted effort on the presented tasks? Did pain, fatigue, diminished arousal, or other factors appear to impede the patient's ability or willingness to perform at potential? Was the patient's approach to tasks linear and goal-directed or did the patient have difficulty staying on task after it was initiated? Were perseverative or impulsive tendencies noted?

To conclude, behavioral observations allow the clinician to summarize initial impressions regarding how the patient thinks, feels, and behaves. In conjunction with these behavioral observations, information obtained through relevant background information (provided by the patient during the clinical interview) creates a context in which objective test scores may be interpreted.

Relevant Background Information

A summary of relevant background information obtained from the patient during the clinical interview further contextualizes objective performances on presented measures. Thorough exploration of key issues from the patient's background serves at least two purposes: (1) identification of historical or current factors that may directly impact the patient's current limitations in functioning, and (2) exploration of the patient's ability to represent his or her background information accurately. Many patients present for neuropsychological evaluation with rather complex and elaborate backgrounds that can be challenging to organize succinctly within the report itself. Clinicians may rely on a structured template that serves to guide the clinical interview and direct organization of the background information section of the neuropsychological report (see Strauss et al., 2006). Some clinicians find it most expedient to question the patient according to the same sequence that is presented within the neuropsychological report.

PRECIPITATING EVENT

One strategy of beginning the background information section is to begin with a summary of the *precipitating event* that may have prompted the referral for neuropsychological evaluation. The precipitating event may represent a stroke, traumatic brain injury, toxic exposure, seizure, or other episode that transpired at a precise point in time. However, the event may also represent a condition or set of conditions that are not easily associated with a particular episode located in time, as in the case of a neurodegenerative process with incipient onset (e.g., Alzheimer's disease), multiple sclerosis, or development of a major depression.

For cases in which the event is clearly identified in time, the background section might begin with a formal statement of when the event took place (e.g., formal diagnosis of Parkinson's disease, time that a stroke transpired). In cases when the event is more difficult to locate precisely in time, it is sometimes helpful to explore the time that a formal diagnosis was offered and then explore the extent to which symptoms either preceded or followed the time of formal diagnosis. Symptoms associated without a clear time of onset can be approximated (e.g., one can simply state that the patient has experienced progressive memory decline for the last approximately three to four years).

Regardless of the ease with which the clinician is able to locate the event in time, a preliminary review of the history surrounding the event—including the onset and course of physical, psychological, and cognitive symptoms that may have coincided with it—can be an effective way of introducing the reader to the event's impact on the patient's current functioning.

ONSET AND COURSE

It is helpful to probe deeply into the patient's understanding of the *onset* and *course* of the cognitive limitation and any ongoing cognitive limitations that the patient may continue to experience. Identification of symptom onset (abrupt, progressive) and course (worsening, improving, stable, fluctuating) may assist the clinician in ascertaining the extent to which the precipitating event(s) may represent a primary etiology, or whether alternative or co-morbid factors might also play a role in the patient's experience of cognitive limitation. In the case of suspected Alzheimer's dementia, for example, it is important to identify whether the symptom onset was relatively incipient and whether there has been progressive memory decline over time. In case of relapsing-remitting multiple sclerosis, the clinician might explore whether the patient's cognitive limitations tend to fluctuate and coincide with flare-up stages of the disease process.

SUBJECTIVE COGNITIVE LIMITATIONS

Detailed exploration of the patient's current *subjective cognitive limitations* is helpful to juxtapose with objective findings. A common complaint among many patients, regardless of etiology, is memory difficulty. In this context, the clinician may ask for specific examples of limitations noted in everyday life. For instance, does the patient experience difficulty recalling recent conversations with a spouse or significant others? If the patient reads the daily paper or other written tracts regularly, has she experienced a diminished ability to retain written forms of information? Are the patient's limitations relevant to more recent (short-term memory) or remote (long-term memory) events? After probing a bit further into the nature of the patient's limitation, it may become apparent that what the patient perceives to be memory difficulty might be more accurately understood as a limitation in attention/concentration. For instance, the patient may complain that he is unable to recollect what a spouse conveys to him in conversation, but with further exploration it is apparent that the greater issue is difficulty in remaining focused during conversations, or while reading, or while viewing television programs. Alternatively, the patient may convey having a memory difficulty recalling the names of familiar acquaintances or family members, and this may raise the possibility that the limitation reflects a dysnomia or other limitation that is language-based.

ACTIVITIES OF DAILY LIVING

After identifying specific examples of the patient's cognitive limitations, it is helpful to identify how these limitations impact the patient's completion of *activities of daily living (ADLs)*. Questions regarding the patient's ability to dress, bathe, and groom can be relevant to older patients. Limitations noted in gait/balance and in handwriting may be explored. The clinician will likely explore the patient's ability to manage finances and pay the bills: Has the patient incurred recent overdrafts or late fees related to cognitive limitations? Has the patient noted changes in his ability to cook or follow recipes? Has the patient left the stove on or water running recently? If the patient continues to work, have others expressed concern about his ability to manage usual duties effectively? What have recent performance reviews or formal evaluations of job performance suggested about her current behavior? Driving is an area of particular importance to explore. Has the patient been involved in recent motor vehicle accidents or received tickets? Has the patient experienced difficulties navigating while driving or become lost in familiar territory? The clinician might also ask whether a spouse or other significant other has expressed concern with regard to the patient's safety while driving.

SOCIAL, ACADEMIC, AND OCCUPATIONAL HISTORY

The clinical interview usually includes information pertaining to the patient's *social, academic,* and *occupational history* to identify pre-morbid factors that may be relevant to current cognitive functioning. It is usually helpful to represent this information chronologically beginning with early development in childhood, and the following questions provide an example of questions that can facilitate efficient identification of key social issues from the patient's background.

- If the patient is aware, was there any history of brain-related trauma during the gestation period or birth process?
- Where was the patient born and raised?
- Was the patient raised by both parents?
- Does the patient have siblings?
- How would the patient describe childhood overall and was there anything unusual about the growing up years (e.g., early abuse)?
- Did the patient show difficulties learning to read, write, or work with numbers in early education?
- Does the patient have any history of learning disability, attention-deficit or hyperactivity, special education, or being held back in school?
- If the patient attended high school, what was the patient's overall grade point average or typical grades?
- What year did he or she graduate?
- Did the patient go on to attend college and graduate school?
- What was the highest degree obtained?
- What is the chronology of the patient's work history?
- Did the patient serve in the military? If so, did he/she face combat? What were the primary duties in service?
- What is the longest job that the patient ever held? How long has the patient been in her/his current position? Does he/she enjoy this position?
- If retired, when?
- Any history of personal injury litigation, workers' compensation or disability claims?
- Has the patient ever been fired?
- Has the patient ever been arrested, imprisoned, or convicted of a crime?
- Has the patient ever married? How many times and how many children?
- Where does the patient currently reside?

FAMILY HEALTH AND PSYCHIATRIC HISTORY

Most clinicians explore in some detail the *family health* and *family psychiatric history*, largely on account of the many conditions that have a strong genetic contribution to the patient's own health history. The clinician may ask whether the patient's parents are living.

- If the patient's parents are deceased, how old were they when they died and what were the causes of death?
- Are the patient's siblings living and how is the health of living siblings?
- Is there any family history of Alzheimer's disease, Parkinson's disease, or other neurologically relevant conditions?
- If there is a history of Alzheimer's disease or other neurologic condition, what was the age of onset (if any) for cognitive manifestations of these conditions?
- Is there a family history of stroke or heart attack?
- In terms of psychiatric history, do any of the patient's family members have a history of formally diagnosed conditions (e.g., depression, anxiety, schizophrenia, bipolar disorder)?
- Is there a family history of substance abuse?
- Is there family history of suicide or self-harming behavior?

PERSONAL HEALTH

A thorough understanding of the patient's *personal health* is essential to the case conceptualization process given the wide range of medical conditions that may potentially impact cognitive, emotional, and behavioral functioning. The personal health history should be explored for history of various medical conditions such as hypertension, hypercholesterolemia, thyroid conditions, stroke, seizure, toxic exposure, and diabetes. Is there a history of traumatic brain injury that resulted in loss of consciousness? If so, the severity of TBI should be explored according to loss of consciousness and duration, post-traumatic amnesia and duration. It may be helpful to inquire as to whether the patient has ever undergone a neurologic examination or neuroimaging study. Has the patient ever been hospitalized and for what reason(s)? Has the patient ever undergone major surgeries? The personal health history may conclude with exploration of any current pain symptoms that the patient may be experiencing (e.g., migraine headaches, back pain). The clinician may gain an understanding of the significance of the patient's pain symptoms by asking him to rate the pain on a scale from one to 10 at the worst and at the best times. How does the patient describe the quality of the pain (sharp, dull, burning, throbbing)? How does the patient treat the pain and is this effective?

PERSONAL PSYCHIATRIC HISTORY

The *personal psychiatric history* should be explored for previous psychiatric hospitalizations, psychiatric consultation, psychotropic medication(s), formally diagnosed psychological conditions, and psychotherapy.

- Has the patient ever experienced self-harming thoughts or exhibited self-harming behaviors?
- Has the patient ever experienced hallucinations ("have you ever seen things or heard things that other people did not see or hear") or delusional thoughts?
- Is there a personal history of alcohol abuse, dependence, or treatment?
- How much alcohol did the patient consume at any given time and for what period of time?
- Does the patient use tobacco or illicit substances?

The personal psychiatric history may conclude with a summary of the patient's current prescribed medications, supplements, and respective dosages.

MOOD AND EMOTIONAL FUNCTIONING

The relevant background information section often concludes with a description of the patient's current *mood* and *emotional functioning*. The clinician might introduce this section by documenting the patient's description of mood within the last few days or weeks.

- Are symptoms and signs of depression or anxiety present?
- Are there indications of major stressors at present (e.g., marital discord, limited financial resources)?
- How does the patient describe his appetite?
- Has her weight been stable within the last month?
- How is the quality of sleep?
- Does the patient feel rested in the morning or experience overwhelming fatigue throughout the day?
- How does the patient enjoy spending his free time (hobbies)?

- Who can she turn to for support (e.g, spouse, friends, family), and is there evidence of sufficient support at the present time?

These areas of the neuropsychological report represent areas that are typically provided by the patient without assistance. However, particularly among patients where there is believed to be greater impairment in everyday life than the patient indicates, it is often helpful to obtain consent to contact an individual familiar with the patient to obtain collateral information pertaining to cognitive and functional considerations.

Collateral Information Provided by Report of Familiar Other

Occasionally, the patient may present for neuropsychological evaluation accompanied by a spouse, parent, child, or other significant other who is familiar with the patient. At other times it is useful for the clinician to obtain the patient's consent to contact a significant other to corroborate information provided during the clinical interview. A summary of a significant other's perspective on the patient's functioning allows the examiner to assess the reliability of self-reported information and obtain an alternative account of how cognitive limitations may or may not impact daily functioning. Relative congruency of accounts between the patient and a significant other may suggest that the patient possesses relatively strong awareness into his or her deficits or limitations (though it should be noted that the significant other may at times have reason to minimize the patient's symptoms, as in the case of a spouse who does not yet have the emotional resources to accept that the patient's memory limitations may be related to a probable Alzheimer's dementia).

Relative incongruity between self-report and information provided by a significant other can provide important information regarding the patient's ability to function in daily life, and may also provide converging information relevant to differential diagnosis (e.g., anosognosia following stroke, diminished insight associated with a frontotemporal dementia, confabulation associated with a Wernicke-Korsakoff syndrome). An interview with a significant other may also be of assistance in providing background information (e.g., medical history) that the patient was unable to provide. Information provided by a significant other can also be compared with information obtained through record review to further understand the patient's background information, though the clinician should also consider the significant other's own ability to provide reliable information about the patient's functioning.

Review of Relevant Available Records

Among patients with relatively complex medical backgrounds, it is usually to the clinician's advantage to identify past or current conditions that are likely to be of relevance to the patient's cognitive functioning. The level of extensiveness in the review process varies according to the context of the evaluation. In most clinical settings, most providers review only those records that are essential to possible brain involvement or medical events that are known to impact cognitive functioning (e.g., review of neuro-imaging test results). In forensic settings, adequate preparation through review of sometimes extensive legal documents in independent medical examinations or other forensic evaluations is key to one's understanding of the chronology of significant events (e.g., when and where a traumatic brain injury may have transpired relative to the onset of the patient's purported cognitive limitations).

Test Results

Presentation of test results according to the cognitive domains discussed in chapter 4 assists the reader in identifying objective data that may (or may not) correlate with the subjective report of cognitive limitation noted by the patient or a significant other. Variations in the presentation of these data are acknowledged. Some clinicians prefer to describe performances in prose only, and then attach a separate summary sheet to the end of the report that depicts standardized (and sometimes raw) score performances broken down by cognitive domain. Others prefer to include descriptions of objective performances and related standardized test results within the text itself. Still others present test scores only and do not provide a description of the tasks themselves.

Summary and Diagnostic Impressions

The examiner often provides a summary of the reason for referral and overview of significant test findings before introducing the diagnostic impressions section. The rationale for a given diagnosis is provided by integration of behavioral observations; information provided through the clinical interview, collateral interview, and record review; and test find-ings. Examiners may incorporate the DSM criteria to arrive at formal diag-noses, but may also rely on alternative diagnostic schemes depending upon which may be deemed to be most clinically beneficial to the patient or referral source. Findings may support both cognitive and psychological diagnoses. At a minimum, the diagnostic impressions section allows the examiner to provide an opinion regarding the following clinical questions:

1. Does the patient show objective evidence of cognitive impairment?
2. What is the extent of impairment (if any)?
3. What potential contributing factors or etiologies may account for the patient's impairments?

The elaborateness of the impressions section varies dramatically according to the requests made by the referral source, the context in which the evaluation transpired (with forensic evaluations usually being far more detail-oriented than clinical evaluations), and the needs of the patient.

Recommendations

If the aim of the impressions section is to identify whether there is objective evidence of cognitive impairment and what factors might underlie that impairment, the aim of the recommendations section is to address the issue of what the findings mean for the patient's functioning in everyday life. An initial recommendation for many patients is to juxtapose the patient's subjective experience of cognitive functioning (whether there is a cognitive complaint or not) with the results of objective testing (whether there is evidence of cognitive impairment or not). If the patient's self-perception is one of significant cognitive limitations, and there is not evidence of cognitive impairment on formal testing, it is possible that anxiety or emotional factors account for the patient's subjective experience of difficulty that may warrant future psychiatric or psychotherapeutic intervention. If the patient's family is concerned about his/her memory functioning and this is denied by the patient but verified on objective testing, the patient's limited insight may play a role in future care needs (e.g., in-home supervision, transition to assisted living).

As in any practice of clinical psychology, it is important to be continually aware that reports have a significant impact on clients' welfare (Ownby, 1997) not only for present purposes that surround the initial clinical referral, but possibly for years to come (Sattler, 1992, p. 726). In consideration of both the patient's cognitive strengths and weaknesses, recommendations that the clinician offers should be simultaneously *realistic* and *practical* (Sattler, 1992). Evidence of relatively mild impairment in learning/memory might prompt a recommendation that the patient consider requesting assistance with everyday tasks that entail the effective management and recall of complex information, such as management of the patient's pharmacologic regimens. For the patient with relatively mild deficits, it might be realistic that the patient maintain some degree of autonomy in these areas of daily living, and it may not be practical or even necessary to have a spouse or loved one uniformly verify that medications are taken on time and as prescribed.

On the other hand, a stronger statement would probably be in order for the patient with more profound disturbance in learning/memory. A realistic statement for this patient might indicate that deficits are significant enough to suggest that the patient should not be expected to manage medications effectively and full support in this area of function is needed. To the extent that this is not practical in the patient's current living circumstances, in-home nursing assistance or transition to a facility that affords such assistance should be considered.

Conclusion

The neuropsychological report is the medium through which the neuropsychologist effectively incorporates various forms of information (e.g., self-report, other report, behavioral observation, relevant records, objective performances) to inform plausible diagnoses, prognoses, and appropriate treatment recommendations. The reader is encouraged to review additional references for further information regarding the art of neuropsychological report writing (Axelrod, 2000; Lezak et al., 2004; Ownby, 1997; Sattler, 1992; Strauss, Sherman, & Spreen, 2006).

PART IV

Other Functional
Competencies—Intervention

SIX

Intervention and Consultation in Clinical Neuropsychology

Intervention in clinical neuropsychology can involve many elements, and neuropsychologists vary widely in the degree to which they participate in activities that are considered to be treatment. The context of the evaluation and subsequent meetings to review results and recommendations are fundamentally clinical activities. Responding to questions and concerns from patients and families is very important and often requires considerable acumen. When done well, a neuropsychological evaluation is an important clinical intervention. The evaluation and follow-up might comprise the only psychologically oriented treatment a patient receives, as in a dementia evaluation. In contrast, the evaluation and feedback session might be the first stage of a more involved therapeutic process involving cognitive rehabilitation, psychotherapy, and interdisciplinary consultation and treatment. While recent surveys indicate little change in reporting of the amount of time neuropsychologists spend treating patients (Sweet et al., 2011; Sweet, Nelson, & Moberg, 2006), there is wisdom in considering interactions with patients as clinical interventions that will impact care decisions and might ultimately benefit the patient in a substantive way.

Given current pressures on reimbursement for diagnostically related services, it seems that provision of therapeutic services might represent a hedge against declining income for neuropsychologists. On one end of the opinion spectrum, Ruff (2003) has suggested that neuropsychologists need to become the "caretakers for cognitive health," and that we are essentially nearing the end of our usefulness as solely clinical diagnosticians. On the other end of the treatment provision spectrum, forensic consultation rarely involves contact that would be considered a therapeutic intervention, though it is certainly a viable source of supplementary income for many neuropsychologists (Kaufmann, 2009; Sweet, Nelson, & Moberg, 2006; Sweet et al., 2011). The stark differences in the kinds of supplementary activities available to neuropsychologists provide some clear choices, though the modal neuropsychologist continues to provide primarily assessment services (Sweet al., 2011; Sweet, Nelson, & Moberg, 2006).

This chapter will briefly discuss circumstances under which neuropsychologists might provide treatment services. As an assessment-oriented profession, neuropsychology has traditionally focused its efforts on diagnosis and consultation. However, the changing practice landscape in professional psychology always affords opportunities to those who might be interested in diversifying their practices. Finally, neuropsychologists' knowledge of the unique concerns of patients with neurobehavioral disorders positions them particularly well to provide treatment services to individuals who are often challenging and misunderstood clinically.

Patient Feedback and Family Consultation

Perhaps the most common intervention-oriented contact that neuropsychologists have with their patients is when they provide feedback regarding assessment results (Gorske & Smith, 2009). In clinical settings this occurs frequently, with more than 70% of surveyed neuropsychologists reporting that they conduct feedback sessions (Sweet, Nelson, & Moberg, 2006). Despite this fact, there is scant literature on this topic, and it is rarely covered formally in internship or postdoctoral fellowships. In contrast, the general clinical literature provides a range of studies focused on using feedback and the interview process as an opportunity to do clinically useful intervention. Perhaps the best known example of this involves motivational interviewing (Rollnick, Miller, & Butler, 2008), which has emerged over the course of the past 20 or so years. It is tempting to draw comparisons with literature on feedback in the general clinical and psychological assessment contexts, though there are clearly differences that make feedback with neuropsychological assessments unique.

Several papers and chapters have addressed the issue of providing feedback, with the focus typically being on what to cover and how to cover it rather than on guiding a specific therapeutic process (e.g., Gass & Brown, 1992; Crosson, 2000). Models based on work presented by Finn and colleagues (Finn & Tonsager, 1992; Finn & Kamphuis, 2006) and Fischer (Fischer 1994; 2003) have described a process wherein the use of psychological assessment results (*not* neuropsychological test results) serves as a platform to encourage needed behavior change. In a recent book, Gorske and Smith (2009) describe their *collaborative therapeutic neuropsychological assessment* approach, which is grounded in basic Rogerian principles. In this model, the patient and neuropsychologist work together throughout the neuropsychological assessment process with a general goal of increasing the patient's understanding of test results and their implications. In doing so, the patient is empowered to make decisions about the treatment process in a collaborative enterprise with the neuropsychologist.

For many traditionally trained neuropsychologists, the notion of "collaborating" with patients might seem jarring. The highly empirical and sometimes detached nature of how neuropsychologists view the assessment process will make this kind of approach a bit of a challenge to warm up to, and would absolutely be seen as inappropriate in forensic neuropsychology settings. For a field that has gained prominence because of its highly empirical approach, a shift to actually using the assessment and feedback sequence therapeutically will likely have its critics and doubters. Nevertheless, few neuropsychologists would object to the notion of using evaluation results to facilitate therapeutic goals (e.g., Gass & Brown, 1992; Crosson, 2000). The extent to which neuropsychologists would use the evaluation as part of a neuropsychologist-driven therapeutic process is also likely to be variable across providers. Assessment contexts are evolving and the realities of changing reimbursement may force neuropsychologists to be more flexible in their views of the nature of their practices. It may be that an extended evaluation process incorporating some manner of intervention could come to meet the standard of being an empirically supported treatment (e.g., Rollnick, Miller, & Butler, 2008) and would ease the burden of proving that the evaluation itself provided adequate value.

Rehabilitation Psychology and Cognitive Rehabilitation

Roughly 12% of neuropsychologist respondents to the 2010 AACN salary survey indicated that their primary place of employment was in a rehabilitation facility. In addition, rehabilitation was the fourth most common institutional department for neuropsychologists (Sweet, et al., 2011), behind psychology, psychiatry, and neuropsychology and slightly ahead of neurology. Presumably, neuropsychologists in rehabilitation settings have experience with a range of interventions used in these settings. Broadly speaking, rehabilitation-based interventions have focused on remediation of specific cognitive deficits and comprehensive rehabilitation programs (Prigatano, 1999; Solhberg & Mateer, 2001; Wilson & Glisky, 2009).

Neuropsychologists have engaged in both specific cognitive interventions (e.g., Cicerone, 2000; Cicerone et al., 2005) and psychological support or psychotherapy (Klonoff, 2010; Prigatano, 2008), both within rehabilitation settings and in outpatient practices. Neuropsychologists have become valued members of the comprehensive rehabilitation team because of their understanding of brain and behavior relationships, assessment-based knowledge, and their contributions to the development of rehabilitation programs.

Early studies in cognitive rehabilitation were often met with skepticism, particularly in neuropsychology circles. However, neuropsychologists have also been a driving force behind research examining the impact of rehabilitation efforts. Many substantive recommendations have emerged from the relatively young cognitive rehabilitation literature, and there is much to be learned in the current climate with its focus on evidence-based practice (Gonzalez-Rothi & Barrett, 2006). Cognitive rehabilitation for specific cognitive deficits has focused on several areas including attention, visuospatial deficits, apraxia, learning and communication deficits, memory, and executive function/problems solving skills (Cicerone et al., 2000; Cicerone et al., 2005; High et al., 2007).

Research examining comprehensive rehabilitation programs has been far less extensive, and the findings have been more difficult to generalize given the nature of the samples and the variable goals of the programs (Cicerone et al, 2005). Nevertheless, there is general interest in outcomes following comprehensive rehabilitation, as evidenced by longstanding funding for model systems programs for spinal cord injury (SCIMS) and traumatic brain injury (TBIMS) through the National Institute on Disability and Rehabilitation Research (NIDRR). These programs are designed to allow longitudinal examination of outcomes for both specific interventions and more broad programmatic interventions. Neuropsychologists involved with these programs have contributed extensively to rehabilitation outcomes research.

While neuropsychologists have been extensively involved in the development of cognitive rehabilitation techniques and treatments, they have not held exclusive domain over such interventions. Colleagues in allied health fields like speech language pathology and occupational therapy are typically responsible for the application of these techniques with inpatients in TBI and stroke programs. Reimbursement for such services is not typically very high; as a result, many neuropsychologists do not view such work as an attractive practice option.

Neuropsychologists in rehabilitation settings are among the first people to assess and appreciate the complexity of issues that confront patients recovering from traumatic brain injury, stroke, and other central nervous system (CNS) affecting disorders. They are often involved in the design and conceptualization of specific interventions and tracking of patient progress. However, the complexity and chronicity of such patients' problems usually require ongoing support and contact with rehabilitation and mental health professionals. Outside of the rehabilitation context, patients continue to need and benefit from interventions that neuropsychologists can provide. This often involves more traditional counseling or psychotherapy, which is the other major category of intervention in which neuropsychologists participate.

Psychotherapy with Cognitively Impaired Individuals

The majority of clinical neuropsychologists are graduates of clinical or counseling psychology doctoral programs (Sweet et al., 2011). Therefore, most are likely to have background and experience with providing psychotherapy services. While surveys indicate that a small percentage of neuropsychologists provide such services, it stands to reason that they would have advantages in understanding the nature of difficulties encountered by cognitively impaired individuals. It is often difficult to find therapists who have experience with brain-injured individuals (Klonoff, 2010; Prigatano 2008), and difficulties can emerge when behaviors and perceptions affected by impaired cognition are misinterpreted by inexperienced therapists.

The focus on empirical data and scientific validation of measures and techniques would seem to equip neuropsychologists well for adding to the growing body of literature on empirically supported treatments (EST) such as cognitive behavioral therapy (CBT; e.g., Anson & Ponsford, 2006), offshoots such as acceptance and commitment therapy (ACT; e.g., Robinson, 2009), and cognitive processing therapy (CPT; e.g., Galovski, & Resick, 2008). Much of this work has been done in the context of polytrauma patients returning from the wars in Iraq and Afghanistan, who have concomitant issues with PTSD and other neuropsychiatric syndromes/disorders (e.g., Chard et al., 2010). Modifications of cognitive behavior therapy have been successful with all manner of patients, but particularly with those struggling with anxiety, depression, and somatoform symptoms (e.g., Bailey et al., 2010).

In addition to CBT based treatments, Prigatano (2008) discusses the importance of understanding and working with underlying psychodynamic issues in individuals with brain injuries. That is, all patients have an important individual developmental history that interacts with how they react and adjust to challenges hastened by their brain injury. While attention to specific cognitive deficits can be fruitful, the complexity and difficulty of adjusting to life with brain impairment exposes many underlying and fundamental elements of an individual's personality and development. As such, a more thorough understanding of dynamic variables can be an asset when treating individuals with long-term psychotherapy. As noted, many neuropsychologists possess unique skills and backgrounds that make them particularly well-suited to offer such services. Whether or not neuropsychologists become more involved in direct treatment and intervention will likely be determined by reimbursement patterns in the future. With health care reform efforts being focused on prevention and primary care, it seems likely that diagnostic services of all kinds will feel pressure to provide evidence of their worth. The extent to which this occurs will inevitably be related to the quality of the evidence base that develops within these specialty areas.

Consultation in Clinical Neuropsychology

CONSULTATION WITH CLINICAL REFERRAL SOURCES (PHYSICIANS, PSYCHOLOGISTS, AND ALLIED HEALTH)

Over the years, neuropsychologists have benefited from a broad referral base, and this has not changed appreciably in recent times. As neuropsychological services became well known to a wide range of professionals, practices in a number of different settings became established (Lamberty, Courtney, & Heilbronner, 2003). Over the past 20 years, neuropsychologists have steadily increased their participation in private practice (Sweet, Moberg, & Suchy, 2000; Sweet, Nelson, & Moberg, 2006; Sweet et al., 2011). The most recent TCN/AACN survey (Sweet et al., 2011) indicates that greater than 50% of all practitioners report some private practice, while the proportion of individuals in sole private practice has increased steadily to somewhere between 25% and 30%. The number of neuropsychologists in institutional-only settings has remained fairly stable at approximately 40% of respondents (Sweet et al., 2011).

Changes from the early days of clinical neuropsychology practice have been considerable with many early practitioners being trained and employed in university hospital-based programs or VA medical centers. Over the years, diversity in practice settings has grown, and this has been noted in various practice surveys (Putnam, 1989; Sweet, Nelson, & Moberg, 2006; Sweet et al., 2011). The range of professionals with exposure to neuropsychological services has probably increased over the years, with neurologists, psychiatrists, physiatrists, psychologists, allied health providers, attorneys, and *independent medical evaluation (IME)* brokers being common referral sources (Sweet, Moberg, & Suchy, 2000; Sweet, Nelson, & Moberg, 2006; Sweet et al., 2011)

The most recent TCN/AACN practice survey (Sweet et al., 2011) indicated different patterns of referrals for neuropsychologists depending upon their practice setting (institution only, private practice only, institution/private practice setting) and their clinical focus (i.e., pediatric, adult, mixed pediatric/adult practices). Table 6.1 shows that across all settings, neuropsychologists received the most referrals from neurology practices, and this did not differ substantially from the previous TCN/AACN

Table 6.1 **Top Five Rankings of Referral Sources Evaluated in Neuropsychological Assessment by General Work Setting and Professional Identity**

	WORK SETTING (GENERAL)		
Rank	Institution only	Private practice only	Institution + Private practice
1	Neurology	Neurology	Neurology
2	Primary care medicine	Law (attorney)[a]	Psychiatry
3	Physiatry	Primary care medicine[a]	Primary care medicine
4	Psychiatry	Pediatrics	Law (attorney)
5	Rehabilitation (rehab nurse, counselor, or other specialist)	Psychiatry	Physiatry

	PROFESSIONAL IDENTITY		
Rank	Pediatric only	Adult only	Pediatric/adult
1	Neurology	Neurology	Neurology
2	Pediatrics	Primary care medicine	Psychiatry
3	School system	Psychiatry	Primary care medicine
4	Self-referral	Physiatry	Pediatrics
5	Other	Rehabilitation (rehab nurse, counselor, or other specialist)	Law (attorney)

Note. Excludes postdoctoral residents.
[a] These factors were endorsed by the same number of participants (i.e., there was a tie).
(Sweet et al., 2011. Reprinted with permission from Taylor and Francis.)

survey. There is variability in the referral sources depending on practitioners' professional identity. For those in adult practice, referrals from psychiatry and primary care practices are common, while pediatric practitioners typically receive more referrals from pediatric practices and school systems. Mixed pediatric/adult practitioners show a mix of those referral sources (i.e., psychiatry, primary care, pediatrics) with attorney referrals rounding out the top five sources. Adult practitioners report more referrals from rehabilitation professionals, while pediatric practitioners receive more self-referrals. Referral patterns as a function of work setting are a bit more comparable, with neurology, psychiatry, and primary care being represented across institutional, private practice, and mixed settings. Legal referrals were common in practices that involve some degree of private practice, while rehabilitation oriented referrals were more common in institutionally based practices.

It seems likely that referral patterns within more specific settings differ from some of these general trends. Some examples might include neuropsychologists practicing within comprehensive epilepsy programs, dementia clinics, or larger psychology/mental health group practices. As economic forces move neuropsychologists to seek employment in more diverse settings, the stability of these referrals also seems likely to change.

CONSULTATION WITH FORENSIC REFERRAL SOURCES (ATTORNEYS, INSURANCE PROVIDERS, AND IME)

A growing referral base in clinical neuropsychology practice involves referrals from the forensic realm including insurance providers, attorneys, and brokers of forensic evaluation services such as independent medical/neuropsychological evaluations (Sweet et al., 2011). Kaufmann (2009) has been a vocal proponent of expanding forensic consulting opportunities given that reimbursement for such services have improved, while other sources of reimbursement (traditional insurance, self-pay) have declined over the past many years. The most recent TCN/AACN survey provides a good deal of information regarding forensic practice patterns and differences in income as a function of the percentage of forensic practice (see Table 6.2; Sweet et al., 2011). There is a clear and positive relationship between income and percentage of forensic practice as well as generally higher levels of job and income satisfaction for those who do some degree of forensic practice. Nevertheless, a substantial minority of neuropsychologists do no forensic practice whatsoever with several groups that are generally less inclined to participate in forensic consultation. Specifically, female

Table 6.2 **Incomes and Frequencies at Various Levels of Forensic Activity**

Forensic activity (%)	n^a	%	Cum %	GROSS PSYCHOLOGY INCOME				
				n^b	%	Mean	Median	*SD*
0	736	49.8	49.8	532	46.1	106.8	95.0	45.0
0.05–19	541	36.6	86.4	462	40.0	138.9	124.0	64.2
20–39	98	6.6	93.0	80	6.9	162.5	149.0	94.0
40–59	50	3.4	96.4	44	3.8	219.2	180.0	158.5
60–79	26	1.8	98.2	20	1.7	232.3	163.0	160.7
80–100	27	1.8	100.0	17	1.5	275.7	200.0	228.7
Total	1478	100.0		1155	100.0	132.5	109.0	80.1

Note.
[a] Excludes postdoctoral residents.
[b] Includes licensed clinicians who work full time or more; excludes postdoctoral residents and income outliers
   (< $33,600). Incomes are expressed in thousands of dollars.
(Sweet et al., 2011. Reprinted with permission from Taylor and Francis.)

practitioners, pediatric neuropsychologists, and those in institutional-only settings report less involvement in forensic practice.

Regardless of these trends, most training programs have not offered specialized training in forensic consulting as part of a customary training sequence. A parallel might reasonably be drawn between forensic consulting services and prescriptive authority, which has been an idée fixe for the APA and other groups over the past twenty or so years (Paige & Robinson, 2003). The argument that psychologists are uniquely equipped to provide medication management services is usually based on the fact that they understand psychopathology and therapeutics in a broad sense, relative to their colleagues in psychiatry, and certainly as compared to those in primary care medicine settings. Therefore, broadening the scope of learning and practice would seem to be a natural form of vertical integration. Similarly, neuropsychologists, with their focus on empirical rigor and knowledge of the neural bases of behavior, should be well equipped to offer expert opinions in the medico-legal context.

Despite the commonsense nature of these assertions, practice in the forensic realm involves an expanded knowledge base and skills that are not typically acquired in the modal graduate training program. Like prescriptive authority, forensic training and consultation is within the realm of most neuropsychologists' ability to learn, and there is no legal prohibition of forensic practice as there is with prescribing medicine. In the current challenging practice climate, the vertical integration of increasingly unfamiliar skill sets has proven to be a popular rallying cry in professional psychology, as it has become in other professions. Whether or not neuropsychologists answer the siren song of broadening forensic roles will likely be determined by many factors. Unfortunately, simply following the money that is often associated with forensic activities can lead to marginal or poor practice in areas that require special focus, additional training, and experience.

Regardless of the foregoing cautions, it is impossible to deny the impact that forensic neuropsychology has had on the general practice of clinical neuropsychology, both in terms of income and contributions to the neuropsychology literature. Sweet et al. (2002) chronicle the impressive growth in forensically oriented offerings in neuropsychology journals in the early part of this century, and Kaufman (2009) suggests that this growth has continued unabated to the present time. Further, forensic neuropsychology has arguably been the most active area of inquiry within neuropsychology, with hundreds of original articles and dozens of texts produced over the past decade (e.g., Sweet, 1999; Larrabee, 2005; Boone, 2007; Heilbronner, 2008). Even with all of these advances and opportunities, neuropsychologists engaging solely in forensic practice are rare, and as noted earlier, many forego forensic practice of any kind (Sweet, Nelson, & Moberg, 2006; Sweet et al., 2011). Thus, while there are many and growing opportunities for neuropsychologists to provide forensic consultation services, this type of practice is adjunctive for most and not necessarily a desirable option for all practitioners.

Teaching/Educational Roles of Neuropsychologists

Neuropsychologists have ample opportunity to work in teaching and educational roles, though the great majority do not work in traditional academic departments. In the recent TCN/AACN survey (Sweet et al., 2011) only 3% of respondents listed the college/university setting as their primary place of employment. However, in the same survey it was found that nearly 17% of the average neuropsychologist's weekly duties involved teaching/training (6.7%), funded research and writing (6.6%), or unfunded research and writing (3.7%). The empirical and data-oriented nature of neuropsychology practice allows for participation in these activities regardless of the settings in which they occur. Indeed, many of the most prolific researchers in clinical neuropsychology work in private practice or other nonacademic settings. Clearly, the opportunity to provide educational services extends beyond traditional academic departments, and neuropsychologists are able to provide such services in a wide range of settings.

In a broader sense, neuropsychologists educate their patients, family members of their patients, and the general public on matters related to a range of conditions they routinely evaluate. In recent times the role of educator has become particularly visible when dealing with the public's concerns about the effects of traumatic brain injury (e.g., McCrea et al. 2008; Gunstad & Suhr, 2001; Mittenberg et al., 2001). In these areas, the expertise and input of neuropsychologists are essential in formulating interventions that fall somewhere between traditional cognitive rehabilitation approaches and individual psychotherapy. As a result, there is a growing body of literature showing that brief, educationally oriented interventions can be very powerful in limiting negative economic outcomes following mild TBI (e.g., Borg et al., 2004). The likelihood that educationally oriented intervention will become increasingly popular seems strong, particularly given pressures to reduce costs of traditional diagnostic and treatment services. The empirical orientation of neuropsychologists positions them well as consultants and providers of psychoeducational services for the many clinical populations that have concerns about cognition and psychological adjustment.

SUPERVISION OF TECHNICIANS, STUDENTS, AND FELLOWS

Neuropsychologists in institutional settings are often involved in some kind of training activity—most often the supervision of students, fellows, and technicians (Stucky, Bush, & Donders, 2010). These activities also occur in other practice settings, though perhaps not in as organized a fashion. The importance of professional supervision cannot be emphasized strongly enough as it is in this context that most neuropsychologists learn the bulk of their clinical trade.

While supervisory activities constitute a small percentage (less than 10%) of the modal neuropsychologist's total work effort in a given week (Sweet, Nelson, & Moberg, 2006; Sweet et al., 2011), those in training settings likely spend considerably more time as supervisors. As noted in chapter 2, training models in neuropsychology have been a focus of the field's professional organizations for many years. The Houston Conference model (Hannay et al., 1998) emerged from the perceived need to have specific aspirational standards for educating and training clinical neuropsychologists, and it has been incorporated as a standard for those seeking board certification in clinical neuropsychology through ABPP/ABCN.

Neuropsychologists have also led the way in establishing a standardized curriculum for postdoctoral training through the Association of Postdoctoral Programs in Clinical Neuropsychology (APPCN; Boake, Yeates, & Donders, 2002). In this context it might seem that there would be equally rigorous and thorough standards for the provision of supervision, but such is not the case. In a recent article, Stucky, Bush, & Donders (2010) outline a model for preparing neuropsychological supervisors that they describe as an "incremental, developmental, and contextual process." The wisdom of such a model is difficult to contest, though the funding for training seems always to be in short supply. Leadership from established programs and organizations will be needed for this kind of model to be implemented beyond a few committed sites.

The TCN/AACN survey has not typically included many items related specifically to supervision, though it does appear that many neuropsychologists engage in some kind of supervisory activity. This may involve basic technical supervision of psychometrists or students, or far more involved supervision of the entire evaluation and feedback process, as might be expected with advanced clinical interns or postdoctoral residents and fellows. More in-depth study of different elements of professional supervision should be a focus of future surveys and studies, as it is often acknowledged as a guiding force in the manner in which professional neuropsychologists practice well into their clinical careers.

PART V

Foundational Competencies

SEVEN

Ethical Standards of Practice in Neuropsychology

We now turn to issues of ethical practice in clinical neuropsychology. The American Psychological Association has published the most consistently relied upon ethical principles of psychologists and code of conduct (APA, 2002). Clinical neuropsychologists, like general practitioners of clinical psychology, rely upon these guidelines more frequently than any other to inform their ethical practices. However, as practitioners of a specialty area, clinical neuropsychologists are also mindful of the generic nature of the APA code and embrace additional resources that are particularly relevant to the practice of clinical neuropsychology. Bush (2007) suggests that in addition to the APA Ethics Code (2002), it is prudent that neuropsychologists familiarize themselves with other published ethics resources, such as edited books (e.g., Bush, 2007), special journal issues on the topic of ethics in neuropsychology (e.g., Bush & Martin, 2006), and other discussions of ethical issues among experienced clinical neuropsychologists (e.g., Johnson-Greene & Nissley, 2008, Bush et al., 2008).

Neuropsychologists are also encouraged to consider the various position papers and policy statements that have been published by professional organizations that are relevant to specified ethical topics. The American Academy of Clinical Neuropsychology (AACN) and the National Academy of Neuropsychology (NAN), for example, have published formal policy statements on various issues such as test security and release of data (NAN; Axelrod et al., 2000; Kaufmann, 2009), informed consent issues (NAN; Johnson-Greene, 2005), the use of non-doctoral level staff in conducting clinical neuropsychological evaluations (AACN, 1999), the presence of third-party observers of neuropsychological evaluations (AACN, 2001), and symptom validity assessment (Heilbronner et al., 2009). Many of these papers can be found at the respective websites of these organizations.

This chapter explores some of the more commonly encountered ethical issues that may arise during neuropsychological evaluation. Topics are presented across three chronological phases: (1) pre-evaluation, (2) evaluation proper, and (3) post-evaluation.

Pre-Evaluation Phase: Ethical Preparation for Neuropsychological Practice

ESTABLISHING THE REFERRAL QUESTION AND ITS APPROPRIATENESS

Prior to the neuropsychological examination itself, it is the neuro-psychologist's responsibility to verify that the examination is clinically indicated or warranted. One factor that complicates this process—for better or worse—is the increasingly high demand for neuropsychological services and limited time that providers have to provide such services. As Attix and Potter (2010, p. 391) state: "clinical neuropsychologists are currently in the midst of a changing health care climate in which reimbursement for services is increasingly linked to definitions of medical necessity, empirically validated treatment, and cost/benefit outcomes." Thus, preliminary consideration of referral appropriateness is prudent for all parties involved for both economic and clinical reasons.

In some work settings, neuropsychologists may feel compelled to honor a request for services related to institutional earnings or productivity expectations. However, the neuropsychologist should never feel obligated to honor a request for services if he or she does not agree that evaluation is clinically indicated. Indeed, one could argue that proceeding with a neuropsychological evaluation that is not perceived to be clinically necessary represents a conflict of interest that could impede one's objectivity in providing services or potentially bring harm or exploitation to the patient (APA Ethical Guidelines 3.05 Avoiding Harm; 3.06, Conflict of Interest).

It may be helpful to consider that requests for services are not static, unidirectional demands placed upon the neuropsychologist by the referral source. Effective triage of referrals entails fluid collaboration and communication with the referral source. Some referring physicians or other providers may have limited experience with neuropsychology and may misunderstand what the evaluation entails. At times, initial referral questions may be vague (e.g., "please assess"), and the clinician should feel free to discuss with the referral source in more detail what expectations informed the request for evaluation. Open communication throughout the referral network can be very helpful in clarifying these issues. A multidisciplinary approach to the referral question maintains the integrity of professional relationships, but more importantly ensures that the patient receives necessary and high quality care.

The neuropsychologist may respond to a referral source's request for services in one of three ways: (1) "yes, let's proceed," (2) "yes, but let's wait," and (3) "no, but let's consider alternatives." Condition (1) is the most common and straightforward scenario. The neuropsychologist determines that the referral question is appropriate and that he or she is capable of providing helpful information to the referral source and patient upon completion of the evaluation.

In condition (2), the clinician perceives that neuropsychological evaluation may be appropriate, but only at a later point in time. As one example, a physician may request that the neuropsychologist identify whether a delirious patient's cognitive limitations may be superimposed upon a dementia without recognizing that a formal diagnosis of dementia cannot be provided in the presence of delirium (DSM). The neuropsychologist may suggest that the patient be evaluated only after the delirium has resolved. As another common example, a physician may desire a dementia screening evaluation in a patient who has a history of untreated sleep apnea. The neuropsychologist may request that evaluation be postponed until the sleep apnea and daytime fatigue have been adequately managed, to gain a "cleaner" understanding of the true source of memory limitations. In scenarios like these, the neuropsychologist takes a pre-emptive step that will aid the eventual case conceptualization process, and, ultimately, better serve the patient.

At other times, such as in the case of condition (3), the neuropsychologist may perceive that neuropsychological evaluation is clearly not warranted based upon what is known of the patient's background or the specific question being asked by the referral source. A physician who refers an actively psychotic individual to rule out ADHD would be a clear example of a referral question that the clinician is unlikely capable of determining, since formal diagnosis of ADHD can be made only to the extent that other Axis I conditions do not account for the patient's symptoms. The neuropsychologist in this situation is encouraged to discuss with the referral source why he or she perceives the evaluation is not appropriate or necessary, and explore alternative outlets for assessment and treatment that are more in line with the patient's limitations and future care needs.

Thus, an essential component of the pre-evaluation phase is determining that the referral question is in fact appropriate, and that the neuropsychologist's provision of services will be of benefit to the patient and other parties with whom the patient is likely to correspond. This process of determining whether to proceed with evaluation can be considered an initial step in providing work that is grounded in scientific and professional knowledge of the discipline (APA Ethical Standard 2.04, Bases for Scientific and Professional Judgments).

COMPETENCE

After the neuropsychologist determines that neuropsychological evaluation is clinically indicated, the clinician should entertain the question: "Am I qualified to do this?" The APA Ethics Code (Standard 2.01, Boundaries of Competence) indicates that psychologists only provide those services that are within the scope of their competence, education, training, and experience. In some clinical environments (e.g., some Veterans Affairs medical centers), guidelines exist to inform whether a clinical psychologist's general background in intellectual or cognitive assessment may be sufficient to conduct brief screens to garner a basic understanding of an individual patient's overall level of cognitive ability. In other circumstances, as in the case of providing services in rural settings (Allott & Lloyd, 2009), it may be possible to provide neuropsychological services to the best of one's ability until a more comprehensive assessment with a more experienced provider can be identified. Ultimately, it is the clinician's responsibility to evaluate the level of competence on a patient-to-patient basis. However, advanced education or background is likely necessary for comprehensive neuropsychological evaluations or to answer more elaborate referral questions.

The most commonly embraced education and training standards for competent practice in clinical neuropsychology are presented by the reports of the INS-Division 40 Task Force on Education, Accreditation, and Credentialing (1987), and the Houston Conference guidelines (Hannay et al., 1998). Under these standards, minimal qualifications to practice neuropsychology include completion of a doctoral degree in clinical psychology or related field, a year of supervised internship training, and two years of postdoctoral training under the direct supervision of a clinical neuropsychologist. Fulfillment of these training requirements typically meets a minimal standard for board certification in clinical neuropsychology, and though not a required element of competency, board certification in the specialty of clinical neuropsychology is becoming recognized as an important marker of competency (Cox, 2010; Johnson-Greene & Nissley, 2008).

Even among seasoned clinical neuropsychologists with the technical competence to proceed with the evaluation, it may be more appropriate to refer to a provider with even greater expertise, depending upon the purpose of the assessment. For instance, an adult neuropsychologist may be competent to address questions related to learning disability or pervasive developmental disorder in a late adolescent patient, but may feel compelled to refer to a pediatric neuropsychologist as available if it is determined that the latter may be even more qualified to provide diagnosis and treatment recommendations. Clinicians with limited forensic experience may feel more comfortable referring an attorney requesting services to a neuropsychologist with more experience in personal litigation or independent medical examination proceedings. In fact, Johnson-Greene and Nissley (2008, p. 954) suggest that "forensic neuropsychological evaluations require specific skills that are typically beyond the average neuropsychologist's expertise." Directing the referral source to other qualified professionals may be the most ethical course of action in these circumstances.

As with all practicing psychologists, it is the neuropsychologist's responsibility to ensure that issues from their personal lives do not interfere with the ability to provide services in a competent manner (APA Standard 2.06; Personal Problems and Conflicts). Medical illness, the death of a loved one, or other life events may impact one's psychological and emotional state, which may in turn diminish the quality of one's professional practice. The standard indicates that when the clinician is aware that personal issues are interfering with their work, that appropriate measures be taken (e.g., consultation with a colleague, limitation or suspension of duties). When providers are aware of a clear conflict of interest that will limit competent practice, appropriate steps are taken to resolve the conflict, most often by referring to another qualified clinician.

Evaluation Proper Phase: Ethical Neuropsychological Practice

INFORMED CONSENT

An initial step to the neuropsychological evaluation is obtaining consent to proceed with the formal assessment. This process is typically completed immediately prior to the clinical interview and often includes presentation of a formal document that summarizes activities associated with clinical neuropsychological evaluation. APA Ethical Standard 3.10 indicates that this process should be completed in language that is reasonably under-standable to the patient. Upon completion of this process, the neuro-psychologist often inquires if the patient has further questions or points of clarification. Some states and federal entities may require only verbal con-sent, but in most circumstances consent is documented via the patient's signature, and the examiner cosigns as the patient's witness to consent.

An important point for the neuropsychologist to emphasize during the informed consent process is that he or she practices within a relational system. In addition to the relationship with the individual patient, the clinician encounters relationships with the referral source (physicians, social workers, attorneys); family members or friends familiar with the patient's level of functioning; insurance carriers that provide reimburse-ment for evaluation; colleagues that may be called upon for consultation purposes; and trainees, psychometrists, and clerks who may have direct contact with the patient. For the neuropsychologist, recognition of these relationships and the various conflicts that may potentially arise from them is an important step to consider during the informed consent process and in upholding ethical practice.

The neuropsychologist discusses with the patient what she or he can expect during and after the evaluation. The clinician emphasizes a commit-ment to maintaining confidentiality (APA Ethical Standard 4.01), but also discusses limitations to confidentiality (APA Ethical Standard 4.02), as in the case of necessary steps to be taken if the clinician perceives that the patient may represent a risk of harming him or herself or others. The clinician discusses who will be interviewing the patient and adminis-tering measures during the assessment phase (e.g., a neuropsychologist, psychometrist). Clarification of the precise role of trainees (if relevant) in neuropsychological evaluation should be provided prior to the neuro-psychological evaluation itself, both to patients and trainees themselves (Stucky, Bush, & Donders, 2010). Issues of disclosure are also discussed (APA Ethical Standard 4.05, Disclosures), and the clinician identifies who will have access to the neuropsychological report (e.g., the patient, referral source, other providers). If administration of measures is to be conducted by support staff other than trainees (e.g., a psychometrist), it is the respon-sibility of the psychologist to ensure that the psychometrist is qualified to conduct assessment techniques (APA Ethical Standard 9.07, Assessment by Unqualified Persons).

In some instances, the patient may not be legally capable of providing informed consent. Children and adolescents usually require the formal authorization of a parent or guardian to proceed with the evaluation.

Martin and Bush (2008) discuss ethical topics specific to work with geriatric patients. Individuals with documented histories of dementia or other incapacitating conditions may have a guardian or other legal appointee who holds power of attorney for health care decisions. In these cases, the clinician should attempt to provide an explanation of the evaluation process, seek assent, and consider the individual's preferences coincident with obtaining the informed consent of the legal guardian (APA Ethical Standard 3.10, Informed Consent). The neuropsychologist should describe the nature and purpose of the assessment services using language that is reasonably understandable to the person being tested (APA Ethical Standard 9.03, Informed Consent in Assessments), even if he or she is unable to technically provide informed consent.

The consenting process is distinct in forensic contexts (e.g., personal injury litigation, disability examination, competency evaluations). When testing is mandated by law, such as in the determination of competency (Moberg & Kniele, 2006), informed consent is typically implied and not usually obtained from the examinee (APA Ethical Standard 9.03, Informed Consent in Assessments). In fact, informed consent in these contexts may be contraindicated since the court, attorney, or other outside entity is the party for whom services are being provided, not the examinee. Nevertheless, the neuropsychologist in these circumstances describes the nature and scope of services provided to the examinee before proceeding (APA Ethical Standard 9.03). For example, prior to the interview and testing sessions, the forensic examiner should discuss with the claimant the referral source (court, attorney, insurance company, employer) the distinctive nature of the examiner's role (i.e., forensic examiner rather than treater), and limitations to confidentiality (e.g., whether an attorney is to receive examination findings).

TEST AND MEASUREMENT SELECTION

As was discussed in chapter 4, the great majority of clinical neuropsychologists employ a flexible battery approach to their assessment practices (Sweet et al., 2011). Test and measurement selection may vary substantially from one provider to the next, and still be deemed ethical practice. However, psychologists are ultimately responsible for the appropriate application, interpretation, and use of assessment instruments that are administered (APA Guideline 9.09c, Test Scoring and Interpretation Services). Further, regardless of the measures employed, the APA Ethical Guidelines clearly present some of the essential qualities of these measures and their benefit to patients. Measures should have known reliabilities and validities

(APA Ethical Guideline 9.02b; Use of Assessments), and should be administered, scored, and interpreted "in a manner and for purposes that are appropriate in light of the research on or evidence of the usefulness and proper application of the techniques" (9.02a). An implicit message of the latter statement is that the assessment measures have established at least a minimal level of empirical support in the published literature.

Psychologists are also directed not to select tests that may be obsolete or outdated to inform intervention decisions or recommendations (APA Guideline 9.08). It should be noted that this standard does not provide explicit direction as to what constitutes an outdated or obsolete test. Additionally, there are instances when a clinician may perceive that an outdated test may be clinically indicated for administration. For patients who have undergone previous neuropsychological evaluation and were assessed with a previous edition of a measure, a clinician may feel that re-administration of the now-outdated test may be in the patient's best interest related to increased ability to identify relative stability or change in cognitive function. As another example, although there have now been two updated editions to the Wechsler Memory Scale (WMS-III, 1997; WMS-IV, 2008) since the publication of the revised edition (WMS-R), many clinician recognize that normative data developed for the WMS-R continue to be preferred in aging patients (Ivnik et al., 1992). In this case it seems that it may be just as ethical—or even more so—to make use of the outdated version of the instrument related to appropriate normative issues.

As another example, when a test publisher develops a subsequent edition of a test (e.g., WAIS-IV, WMS-IV), is it the clinician's responsibility to begin administering the updated revision immediately after test release? Bush (2010) discusses this very issue. He notes that while the presumed intention of test revision is to improve upon psychometric properties and normative data of previous editions, consensus regarding *when* to begin administering the updated measure has not been established; neuropsychologists may have good reason to delay administration of updated versions of tests. He states that "it often takes years after publication of a new version of a test for research with special patient populations to be performed and published, and even then the findings may not reveal superiority of the newer version of the test for use with certain populations" (p. 8). The clinician may feel that continued use of previous editions may be the best course of action until convergent literature confirms the appropriate use of updated measures in specific populations. Bush (2010) concludes that the final decision to adopt a test revision is at the clinician's discretion; the decision "should be based on the clinician's informed professional judgment after careful consideration of the specific needs of the practice setting and patient whose neuropsychological functioning is being evaluated" (p. 14).

APA Ethical Guideline 9.02b (Use of Assessments) emphasizes the importance of using measures with known reliability and validity information "with members of the population tested." In cases when a patient's background may be different from published normative data, the clinician describes the strengths and limitations of test results and interpretation. Strengths and limitations of conventional assessment instruments in diverse ethnic and cultural groups, whose backgrounds and languages may differ substantially from patient groups on which normative data are based, are especially important for the clinician to consider when interpreting neuropsychological findings.

Cultural and Diversity Issues. In the context of the rapidly changing cultural, ethnic, and racial makeup of Western society, neuropsychologists are more and more likely to face the challenges of assessing patients whose backgrounds may not typify the normative samples (usually Western) against which individual test performances are conventionally rated. As such, there is great need to increase the cultural competence of clinical neuropsychologists (Mindt et al., 2010). Social, cultural, racial, and ethnic factors have been shown to account for significant performance variability on standardized neuropsychological measures (Brickman, Cabo, & Manly, 2006; Romero et al., 2009). Language acquisition, quality of education in one's native culture, and acculturation are examples of factors that may impact performances on cognitive measures. Faced with these potential confounds, the neuropsychologist may be unable to conclude whether impaired performances reflect underlying brain dysfunction, or are more likely attributable to psychometric limitations of measures when administered to culturally diverse clientele.

APA Ethical Standard 9.06 (Interpreting Assessment Results) indicates that psychologists should "take into account the purpose of the assessment as well as various test factors, test-taking abilities, and other characteristics of the person being assessed, *such as situational, personal, linguistic, and cultural differences that might affect psychologists' judgments or reduce the accuracy of their interpretations* (emphasis added)." However, while the standard suggests that the psychologist take cultural factors into account, it does not provide specific guidance as to *how* psychologists should most effectively accomplish this. In fact, establishing effective and ethical practices in culturally diverse populations has been the topic of a rather substantial cross-cultural neuropsychology literature in recent decades. A theme of this literature is that cultural factors clearly matter when interpreting performances, but that ongoing research is clearly needed to inform best practices when working with culturally diverse patients.

Brickman, Cabo, and Manly (2006), for example, highlight the complexities of working with cross-cultural patients, and emphasize the need for future discussions and research in test selection and development. The authors cite various studies showing that minority samples tend to underperform relative to normative Caucasian samples, even after controlling for key demographic variables such as education. The authors emphasize that it would be inaccurate to conceive of race or ethnicity in and of themselves as causing variability in test performances. Rather, race and ethnicity can be understood as markers for various factors such as level of acculturation, which may in turn impact cognitive performances. The authors emphasize the importance of developing and refining measures to improve assessment accuracy and to "inform overarching questions about valid measurement of cognitive ability, regardless of diversity matters" (p. 98).

The issue of evaluating patients who speak English as a secondary language or not at all is commonly encountered by neuropsychologists and warrants comment. APA Ethical Guideline 9.02 (c) (Use of Assessments) states that "psychologists use assessment methods that are appropriate to an individual's language preference and competence, unless the use of an alternative language is relevant to the assessment issues." To the extent that the neuropsychologist has familiarity with the patient's individual cultural background and language, it is possible to conduct the assessment in the native language of the patient. However, many neuropsychologists do not possess the necessary bilingual (or multilingual) skills or cultural familiarity to conduct such evaluations themselves.

In these circumstances, neuropsychologists sometimes opt to evaluate patients in conjunction with an interpreter. APA Ethical Standard 9.03 (c) indicates that when psychologists rely upon an interpreter to obtain test results, they discuss limitations of the data obtained. However, the practice of relying upon the services of an interpreter in neuropsychological evaluation of patients who do not speak English as a primary language is controversial. Some have recommended against using interpreters, related to limited research showing that this is psychometrically justified. Artiola i Fortuny (2008, p. 968) states: "As far as I know, research on the consequences of the use of interpreters in neuropsychology does not exist." However, consensus on this issue has not been established. It is our recommendation that clinicians conduct a detailed cost-benefit assessment when considering relying on the services of an interpreter, and then proceed only when it is determined that it would be of greater harm to the patient not to proceed.

Issues of culture and diversity will continue to be important for neuropsychologists to consider in their clinical and research practices for years to come. In the context of this increased need, Romero et al. (2009) summarize proceedings of a Multicultural Problem Solving Summit that was convened at the annual meeting of the International Neuropsychological Society (INS) in February 2008. The primary aim of the summit was to plan for the future of cross-cultural neuropsychology and identify specific targets to be considered for future research. Summit participants included experienced neuropsychologists, test publishers, trainees, and younger neuropsychology professionals who were there to gain multiple perspectives on ethnically based norms, research and scientific approaches, and an appropriate education and training in multicultural neuropsychology. Efforts like these play an essential role in formulating the future of ethical practices in culturally diverse samples.

THE NEUROPSYCHOLOGICAL REPORT

Just as test selection may vary substantially from one provider to the next and still be deemed ethical practice, the style and format of the neuropsychological report may vary and still be considered an appropriate method of summarizing patient information and test results. As discussed in chapter 4, a great deal of variability exists in report writing style among clinical neuropsychologists (Donders 2001a, b). Nevertheless, the APA Code (2002) includes guidelines that should be considered during the report writing process.

Ethical standard 2.04 indicates that psychologists' work be based upon established scientific and professional knowledge of the discipline. This again speaks to the importance of making interpretations that are grounded in the empirical literature as a whole to inform plausible diagnoses and appropriate treatment recommendations for the individual patient. Ethical standard 9.01a (Bases for Assessments) further indicates that psychologists provide only those that are sufficient to substantiate their findings. When clinicians are unable to conduct an examination that is adequate to support their statement or conclusions, they clarify the potential impact of limited information and "appropriately limit the nature and extent of their conclusions or recommendations" (9.01b).

An important factor for neuropsychologists to consider when generating reports is that not all information conveyed during a clinical interview need necessarily be included in the report itself. In keeping with Ethical Guideline 4.04 (Minimizing Intrusions on Privacy), the neuropsychologist typically discusses background information that may be relevant to cognitive function, the ability to maintain activities of daily living, and other information that may be important to consider when offering treatment recommendations. In so doing, the neuropsychologist appropriately includes "only information germane to the purpose for which the communication is made" (4.04a).

As a rule of thumb, the clinician should report information in a way that he or she would feel comfortable conveying to the patient face-to-face. Clinicians should be mindful that patients typically have the right to request access to most forms of information obtained during the clinical neuropsychological evaluation, including the neuropsychological report. It is also important to recognize that other psychologists or patient providers may have access to the report, which further highlights the importance of practicing discretion when considering how to describe evaluation results.

Post-Evaluation Phase: Ethical Practice Following Neuropsychological Evaluation

RELEASE OF INFORMATION

Upon completion of the neuropsychological evaluation, the neuropsychologist considers who will have access to evaluation results. Typically, the clinician identifies who will have access to evaluation results during the informed consent process. The neuropsychologist may receive subsequent requests from the patient to release information to outside parties. This request should be honored only after a release has been signed by the patient or the patient's guardian, as necessary.

In addition to the neuropsychological report itself, APA Standard 9.04a indicates that neuropsychologists are to release test data to the patient or other individuals as requested by the patient, and Standard 9.04b indicates that in the absence of patient release, psychologists provide test data only as required by law. There are exceptions to this. APA Standard 9.04a indicates that psychologists may refrain from releasing test data to protect the patient from substantial harm. In the case of a patient who is identified as having probable Alzheimer's disease, for example, the clinician may perceive that the patient may not have the ability to understand the nature and implications of test findings, and decide to withhold findings in the interest of reducing harm to the patient. In this scenario, the clinician may request the patient's permission to convey results to a family member or other individual to ensure that test results are used appropriately (e.g., to inform treatment planning) before discussing evaluation results with the patient.

Disclosure of neuropsychological test data has been a topic of extended discussion in recent years (Attix et al., 2007; Axelrod et al., 2000; Bush & Martin, 2006; Kaufmann, 2009). Much of this dialogue has centered upon the noteworthy distinction between *test data*, which in most circumstances a patient has the right to obtain, and *test materials*, which the patient does not have the right to obtain. According to the APA Code (2002), test data include raw scores, standard scores, patient responses to test items (not the items themselves), and the clinician's notes. Many clinicians include raw and standard scores as an addendum at the end of the neuropsychological report, and as a result the patient would have access to these scores simply by requesting access to the report itself.

In contrast, APA Standard 9.11 (Maintaining Test Security) describes test materials as referring to manuals, instruments, protocols, test questions, or stimuli, and does not include test data as defined in Standard 9.04. The same standard indicates that "psychologists make reasonable efforts to maintain the integrity and security of test materials and other assessment techniques consistent with law and contractual obligations, and in a manner that permits adherence to this Ethics Code."

There are at least two reasons why it is essential for neuropsychologists to maintain the security of test materials. First, test manuals, instruments, and stimuli, are typically copyrighted forms of information and the property of the test development companies. Unauthorized release of test materials to non-psychologists is likely to violate copyright laws. Second, the effectiveness of standardized measures is to a significant extent related to the novelty of their content. When test content is made available to the test-taker prior to evaluation, reliability and validity of those results may be profoundly compromised. Protection of test security is protection of the public's interests. As Axelrod et al. (2000, p. 383) state: "maintaining test security is critical, because of the harm that can result from public dissemination of novel test procedures."

Attix et al. (2007) note that the issue of releasing test data may vary according to state law, federal law, and Health Insurance Portability and Accountability (HIPAA) requirements. They provide a helpful flowchart to assist the clinician in navigating conflicts that may exist between these legal entities and the APA Ethics Code. They note, for example, that the clinician may in some circumstances be required to release testing protocols on which patient responses were provided, as it may not be possible to separate test items from respective responses (e.g., when direct responses are recorded on a WAIS-III record form). In ambiguous situations like these, it is suggested that neuropsychologists consult with an attorney or other qualified individuals to clarify state and federal law requirements and guide appropriate action (Bush & Martin, 2006).

FEEDBACK

The final component of the neuropsychological evaluation involves provision of feedback to the patient, family, referral source, or others who may have interest or clinically driven need for evaluation findings. As described by APA Ethical Standard 9.10 (Explaining Assessment Results), psychologists "take reasonable steps to ensure that explanations of results are given to the individual or designated representative unless the nature of the relationship precludes provision of an explanation of results." Examples of the latter scenario include forensic examinations in which the claimant or examinee is not the designated patient and test results are likely to be communicated to disability insurance carriers, attorneys, or other outside parties.

In many circumstances, the feedback session can be a very meaningful time for patients and their families. A clinician's conclusion that a patient's subjective experience of memory limitation is age-appropriate may come as some relief for certain aging patients. Even among patients who show significant limitations in function that are believed to be consistent with early stage of Alzheimer's or dementia, the patient or family may find the results to be verification of the observations made in daily life.

Provision of feedback can be more challenging when test results are not clearly congruent with some of the personal experiences that are described by the patients or their families. Even more difficult is the issue of providing feedback to patients who demonstrate insufficient effort or response invalidity following neuropsychological evaluation (Carone, Iverson, & Bush, 2010). In these situations, neuropsychologists are encouraged to consider how to maintain the integrity of test findings while also balancing the concerns that the patient may have about these findings. Similar to the work of clinical psychologists who conduct general assessment activities (e.g., Finn & Tonsager, 1997), the neuropsychologist is encouraged to identify strategies of making test results therapeutic and beneficial to patients and their families.

Conclusion

Published works pertaining to ethics in neuropsychology has proliferated in recent years. This trend seems to coincide with the continued solidification of neuropsychology as a distinct specialty area of practice. The reader is strongly encouraged to consult these many references for additional information. This chapter has highlighted just a few ethical issues that are encountered by neuropsychologists in routine practice, and it is hoped that discussion of these issues will inspire the clinician to be continually mindful of ethical issues and to maintain high quality care of the patients that we evaluate.

EIGHT

Future Directions

In chapters 1 and 2 we discussed the evolution and growth of clinical neuropsychology and noted that our field has evolved impressively over the past 40 years. In the latter half of the twentieth century, these gains were made in a general health care environment that valued scientific inquiry and fostered the growth of clinical science and innovation. However, expenditures on health care, related disciplines, and associated scientific endeavors over the past 50 years were enormous and unsustainable. Debates about how to manage care have been common since the early 1990s and various proposed solutions (e.g., HMOs, PPOs, MCOs) have not provided a clear fix for escalating costs and the ability to provide care to growing numbers of uninsured or under-insured individuals. In March 2010, the Affordable Care Act (see http://www.healthcare.gov) was signed into law with changes that promised to be wide-ranging. The size and complexity of the law make it difficult to know the exact extent to which changes will occur for various clinical fields and practitioners. Further, changes in the composition of the U. S. Congress in late 2010 suggest that the debate and uncertainty about the full enactment of the Affordable Care Act will continue. Therefore, in today's health care climate it seems certain that proposed changes in public law and resulting reimbursement policy and practices will have an impact on nature of most clinical practices.

The practice of clinical neuropsychology *is* being impacted by changes in health care policy, but dissatisfaction with managed care and reimbursement practices has been present for many years (Sweet, Westergaard, & Moberg, 1995; Kanauss, Schatz, & Puente, 2005). Neuropsychologists have used a variety of strategies to adapt their practices to changes in reimbursement, including not accepting insurance (self-pay), varying the mix of their payors, changing the nature of services they offer, and increasing the amount of forensic consultation that they do. Still, business as usual will inevitably change, and the success of neuropsychology and its practitioners will depend upon a nimble and informed approach to changes in the health care landscape. In the past, it has generally been the case that the value of neuropsychological services was accepted by referral sources and third-party payors, but this state of affairs will no longer be enough to insure adequate reimbursement for neuropsychological services.

The foremost challenge for the field of clinical neuropsychology in upcoming years will be to demonstrate the value of neuropsychological services. There are a number of ways to approach this challenge, many of which were discussed in a special issue of *The Clinical Neuropsychologist* focusing on Advocacy in Neuropsychology (Volume 24, Number 3). Ideally, advocacy for successful practice and what is ultimately best for patient care should not be markedly different, but the standard for proving this is becoming increasingly evidence-based. Early notions of evidence-based practice in medicine have been around for 20 or more years (Evidence-Based Medicine Working Group, 1992), and have taken a bit longer to catch on in the broader practice of psychology (APA, 2006; Chelune, 2010). However, with an increasing number of health care practitioners competing for a presumably declining amount of health care funding, decisions made on political and scientific fronts will dictate the future of our field. This final chapter will discuss ways that neuropsychology and neuropsychologists can help ensure that they are not marginalized as health care goes through inevitable changes. Successful maintenance of the field's stability in the current economic landscape will be accomplished only through ongoing efforts to conceptualize professional identity, establish active and fruitful advocacy practices, and demonstrate an empirical evidence base that neuropsychological services are in fact cost effective and beneficial to patients.

Professional Identity

One of the most important strategies of maintaining the credibility of clinical neuropsychology—as well as its marketability—is to continually develop explicit criteria that inform professional identity. Development of criteria supporting eligibility for board certification in clinical neuropsychology is an example of how the field has shaped professional identity over the years. In chapter 2, we discussed neuropsychology's development as a clinical and professional field. This growth has been mostly positive, but challenges have existed in determining the most appropriate and positive direction for the field. Over the past many years a number of different groups have shown interest in moving the profession forward by increasing opportunities for practitioners. The debate about how this is best done has been contentious and has sometimes degenerated into squabbling about fairness, elitism, and restraint of trade. In one instance, a statistical analysis of board certification trends suggested that it was "conceivable that improperly rejected applicants and even those who have never applied might complain that ABCN is interfering with various rights associated with practicing one's profession, free trade, competition in the marketplace, and so forth. False rejection can permanently undermine a professional's credibility, reputation, and income" (Rohling, Lees-Haley, Langhinrichsen-Rohling, & Williamson, 2003; pg 346). In reality, the trends noted in that particular article have not continued, and ABCN has certified more specialists than has any other ABPP board (or any non-ABPP neuropsychology board). Figure 8.1 shows the historical increase in individuals having achieved board certification through ABCN. The total number of diplomates awarded doubled between 1998 and 2009. It took 18 years (1981–1997) to reach that number from the time the board was established. Figure 8.2 shows the trend in the number of individuals becoming board-certified on a yearly basis. From 1993 through 2001, an average of 25.2 individuals were certified yearly, while 37.2 per year were certified between 2001 and 2010. This is an increase of approximately 48% yearly during these consecutive epochs of time. Over the past 5 years the trend has continued to grow, with 44 newly certified ABCN diplomates a year. Regardless of the progress made, it continues to be the goal of

FIGURE 8.1 **Inclusive Number of ABCN Diplomates in Clinical Neuropsychology over Time**

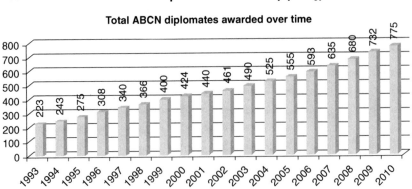

FIGURE 8.2 **Number of ABCN Diplomates in Clinical Neuropsychology on a Yearly Basis**

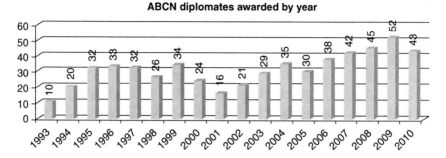

ABCN to establish board certification as a standard for practicing neuropsychologists. The capacity for examining and certifying new diplomates will most certainly need to grow to keep up with the trends seen in the past several years.

In fairness, the article by Rohling, Lees-Haley, Langhinrichsen-Rohling, & Williamson (2003) may have served as a catalyst for ABCN to make information about their process more accessible and encouraged ongoing revision of their examination protocol. The ABCN Board continuously updates and modifies their process with the goal of being responsive to the needs of the profession and its practitioners. It is clear that board certification in psychology has not yet achieved the kind of recognition and penetration that board certification has attained in medicine, but ABCN and AACN's successes in the past decade have served as a model for other ABPP Boards and Academies (Cox, 2010). Practically speaking, board certification through ABCN has begun to show decided benefits of a kind that should stimulate continued growth. Cox (2010) mentions several potential benefits of board certification including potential for higher income, decreased malpractice liability costs, streamlined licensing, increased practice mobility, demonstration of program credibility, increased job satisfaction and marketability, reduction in public confusion, and the consolidation of skills learned throughout the career. Armstrong et al. (2008) also highlight many benefits of ABCN certification in their primer on the process. These sources are clearly advocates for the ABCN board certification process, but they also highlight the reality of a high level of organization and effort that has gone into promoting a process that many believe should ultimately become a standard in the field (e.g., Bieliauskas, 1999). Finally, the TCN/AACN surveys have consistently shown a positive association between board certification through ABCN and income, income satisfaction, and job satisfaction (Sweet, Nelson, & Moberg, 2006; Sweet et al., 2011).

Despite potentially distracting and negative debates about credentialing processes, board certification through ABCN has provided a solid credential and the ability to identify oneself as a neuropsychologist committed to a high level of practice. Further, the American Academy of Clinical Neuropsychology has developed a wide range of benefits for its board-certified specialists and the field at large including its popular journal, a critically acclaimed book series, a growing CE-based annual conference, and informative list serves. Rather than wallowing in internecine bickering, these groups have forged ahead with initiatives that advocate for neuropsychologists in legislative and legal processes, help them with marketing their practices, and improve their visibility among their colleagues.

Arguments about exclusivity and elitism will continue to be raised by those who do not avail themselves of the benefits of board certification, or who see the process as draconian. Detractors of the process are known to lament the lack of hard evidence that board certification is a guarantee of anything, or perhaps that there is an inherent unfairness or irrelevancy in the standards used to certify competence. The alternative is to make certification essentially meaningless by promulgating standards that can be claimed by nearly anyone. In the end the market will decide, and that market is becoming increasingly dominated by those who put themselves up to the scrutiny of a process like that of the ABCN.

Advocacy

The notion of advocating for one's professional interests seems to inspire a spectrum of opinions. On the too-typical end of the spectrum, advocacy might be associated with shilling or pandering. Spending time and money on convincing others of one's worth is fundamentally unseemly. If what we do is worthwhile, that value should be self-evident, with the work product being the only advocacy that is needed. Such a view is logically appealing, but practically naïve. On the other end of the philosophical spectrum, advocacy is seen as a way to secure a place at the table, and no level of effort is irrelevant or excessive. In both cases, the would-be advocate might believe steadfastly in what it is he or she has to offer, though this is not as clear from the non-advocating end of the spectrum.

Today's health care landscape is convoluted and often driven by legislative actions that seem far removed from the clinical settings in which services are delivered. Policy set by the Centers for Medicare and Medicaid

Services (CMS) establishes reimbursement rates for the federal health care programs, as well as serving as a guideline for insurers in the private sector. The mix of individuals and groups that are responsible for determining reimbursement rates is equally complex and rarely involves psychologists or neuropsychologists. As noted by Howe, Sweet, & Bauer (2010), "most critical decisions that affect neuropsychological practice are made by non-neuropsychologists" (p. 375), underscoring the importance of involvement of neuropsychologists on many different levels of legislative and professional affairs.

Neuropsychologists are clearly frustrated by the state of managed care and the limited amount of reimbursement that they receive for their services. In a survey of the National Academy of Neuropsychology (NAN) membership, Kanauss, Schatz, and Puente (2005) found that nearly 78% of respondents either had a negative or negative/neutral opinion of managed care. Judging by the amount of time that was required of the sample to complete evaluations and the percentage of time that was actually approved for services, this dissatisfaction seems quite understandable. For example, respondents in the study reported that forensic evaluations took approximately 10 hours to complete, whereas the percentage of the original amount billed that was approved for reimbursement was averaged only 95 minutes.

Furthermore, securing reimbursement for specific cohorts, such as geriatric patients under Medicare (Jamora, Ruff, & Connor, 2008), or in certain school districts in the case of educational exams (Ernst, Pelletier, & Simpson, 2008), can be especially limited and may preclude neuropsychologists from evaluating these individuals. If neuropsychologists are frustrated by these circumstances, it is suggested that they consider strategies by which they might assist in advocating on behalf of the field to effect change.

Howe, Sweet, and Bauer (2010) make several recommendations about how neuropsychologists can become more involved in professional advocacy, including educating the general public and other practitioners about what neuropsychologists do, becoming more involved in political activities that impact neuropsychology practice, and supporting APA and neuropsychology organizations. As with many things, knowing oneself is important in determining how to best support and advocate for your profession. Doing nothing seems particularly shortsighted and likely to result in substantial changes in how neuropsychology practice is conducted.

Competition for health care reimbursement and grant funding is intense, and funding decisions sometimes appear capricious. Over the years, neuropsychology organizations have had variable success in working with

other professions, and this has resulted in some favorable recommendations about how neuropsychological assessment fits into the larger care and
management picture for specific patient groups (e.g., Petersen et al., 2001).
Equally often—or perhaps more frequently—neuropsychology has found
itself on the outside looking in on these processes. The major neuropsychology organizations (AACN, APA D40, and NAN) have increasingly
responded to some of these situations with position papers and statements
underscoring the value and importance of neuropsychological services.
This is a common strategy to help inform the public, though it is clearly
limited in the sense that is unidirectional. That is, a guild organization provides information about its services to whoever might be interested. What
is lacking in that situation is any sort of reciprocal communication or the
ability to persuade decision makers that neuropsychology should be an
integral part of patient care.

Relationships with other organizations and specialties can be difficult to
establish and maintain, and it is also difficult to quantify how beneficial a
given relationship is. Too often, professional neuropsychology has seemed
to err in its confidence that it would be regarded as important without
reaching out to colleagues in allied disciplines. There seems to have been
some professional xenophobia in the past, and this is increasingly problematic when feedback from organized neuropsychology is not sought on
important matters. By way of example, in late 2010, three different situations arose in which practitioners of neuropsychology might have been
substantially impacted:

- First, the Social Security Administration (SSA) put forth proposed
  rules for evaluating disability claims secondary to mental disorders.
  While several proposed changes were positive for psychology, other
  parts of the language did not clarify the nature of assessments to be
  conducted or the properties of the measures to be used. Since this is in
  the domain of neuropsychologists' unique experience and expertise,
  the AACN and APA Division 40 crafted a response recommending
  more specific language and also provided commentary related to
  populations and tests that neuropsychologists routinely employ (http://
  www.theaacn.org/position_papers/AACN_response_to_SSA.doc).

- In another situation, the American Medical Association's (AMA)
  Physician Consortium for Performance Improvement (PCPI)
  requested public commentary on a dementia performance
  measurement set, and it was clear that their group had no
  representation from organized neuropsychology. The AACN sent a

letter recommending consideration of more specific neuropsychological measures, as well as offering to become part of the consortium in future endeavors (http://www.theaacn.org/position_papers/AACNresponse_to_AMA_PCPI_Dementia_Performance_Measurement_Set.pdf).

- Finally, concern was expressed about the potential negative effect that the state of Minnesota's policies pertaining to neuropsychological services might have for practitioners of neuropsychology (http://www.theaacn.org/position_papers/AACN-ABCN-ResponseToMN.pdf). Ironically, the State of Minnesota recommended that only ABCN certified neuropsychologists would be approved for reimbursement of neuropsychological services. The ABCN and AACN Boards responded with their recommendations to provide a workable solution to this issue, while still advocating for the ABCN board certification process (http://www.theaacn.org/position_papers/AACN-ABCN-ResponseToMN.pdf). Again, an offer to partner with the State of Minnesota was extended, and this sort of collaborative effort will be essential for neuropsychology to continue to be a force within organized health care.

There are few neuropsychologists practicing in the United States compared to the number of practitioners in other disciplines. Therefore, no matter how strong our science or helpful our clinical insights, alliances with other professionals are essential to our future economic survival. A strategic approach would be to attend to our most common referral sources including neurology, psychiatry, primary care, and rehabilitation medicine (Sweet, Nelson, & Moberg, 2006, Sweet et al., 2011). Cooperating on an organizational level with these professions might improve prospects and at the very least visibility when intradisciplinary efforts are requested.

Evidence-based Practice and Focus on Outcomes

Following the recent sociopolitical trends that have emerged in the area of health care reform in the United States, clinical psychologists and neuropsychologists alike have faced the challenge of essentially proving that the services they provide are beneficial to their patients. This seems quite reasonable, given the limited resources that are available. In the general field of clinical psychology, the result has been development of evidence-based intervention approaches that, for better and for worse, have defined much of the current culture of therapeutic practice. For general practitioners, the emphasis on empirically based practice has not met with uniform satisfaction. Some have seriously questioned the assumption that empirically supported treatments necessarily connote greater evidence of being therapeutically beneficial, or that they are necessarily more deserving of reimbursement. Wachtel (2010, p. 254), for example, suggests that manualized therapies have "increasingly become a *requirement* by granting agencies for funding research, and training in 'manualized treatment' has become widely (and falsely) equated with training in therapeutic approaches that are based upon solid and reliable evidence."

Neuropsychologists, too, have faced increased need to demonstrate that their practices are evidence-based. Generally, however, neuropsychologists are only just beginning to discuss and research the topic of evidence-based practice. Drawing from key elements outlined in the broader realms of evidenced-based medicine (EBM; Sackett et al., 2000) and evidence-based psychological practice (EBPP, APA Presidential Task Force, 2006), Chelune (2010) provides suggestions for an evidence-based clinical neuropsychological practice (EBCNP). He recommends that developing this evidence base will rest upon the ability of neuropsychologists to clearly define outcomes that can be applied by clinicians. For example, regular consideration of base-rate information and classification accuracies (e.g., false positives, false negatives, odds ratios) may support relevant outcomes that allow payers to determine the value of neuropsychological services.

In response to the call for evidence-based practice, the American Academy of Clinical Neuropsychology (AACNF; http://aacnf.org/) has recently established the Outcome Measurement Grant Committee, which solicits proposals for funded research that directly examines the evidence base of neuropsychological outcomes. The first award was granted to a proposal examining the applicability of neuropsychological services in reducing the use of medical resources. It is hoped that endeavors like these will serve as a springboard for further research showing the benefits of neuropsychological services in medical and other assessment settings.

In the context of innovations made in neuroimaging, completion of the human genome project, advances in information science, and the current state of health care, Bilder (2011, p. 8) argues that the field of neuropsychology is currently "poised for a paradigm shift." Although satisfactory achievement of this shift will likely require years of commitment, Bilder argues that there are various actions that neuropsychologists can institute at the present time "to accelerate change and prepare for the future" (p. 9). Continued formulation of the concepts that underlie our measures, development of innovative assessment approaches, and large-scale collaboration are examples of steps that will need to be taken to ensure that the field continues to evolve.

This is a very exciting time in the history of clinical neuropsychology. The field has clearly flourished since its inception decades ago, and we perceive that the field will continue to progress in the years to come. However, there is little doubt that the field is currently at a crossroads. The field's future success will only be assured to the extent that neuropsychology clinicians and researchers are willing to clarify and demonstrate its merits. Paradigmatic shifts are inevitable in any scientific field, and neuropsychology is no exception. It is sometimes tempting to become discouraged by the recent challenges that have thwarted the status quo. It may be more adaptive to conceive of these as opportunities to be taken to the benefit of our practices, and ultimately, to the patients we serve.

Reports of the INS/Division 40 Task Force on Education, Accreditation, and Credentialing

Text reprinted with permission from Taylor & Francis.
INS–Division 40 Task Force on Education, Accreditation, and Credentialing. (1987). Report of the INS–Division 40 Task Force on Education, Accreditation, and Credentialing. *The Clinical Neuropsychologist, 1,* 29–34.

Reports of the INS/Division 40 Task Force on Education, Accreditation, and Credentialing

Guidelines for Doctoral Training Programs in Clinical Neuropsychology

Doctoral training in Clinical Neuropsychology should ordinarily result in the awarding of a Ph.D. degree from a regionally accredited university. It may be accomplished through a Ph.D. programme in Clinical Neuropsychology offered by a Psychology Department or Medical Faculty or through the completion of a Ph.D. programme in a related specialty area (e.g., Clinical Psychology) which offers sufficient specialization in Clinical Neuropsychology.

Training programmes in Clinical Neuropsychology prepare students for health service delivery, basic clinical research, teaching, and consultation. As such they must contain (a) a generic psychology core, (b) a generic clinical core, (c) specialized training in the neurosciences and basic human and animal neuropsychology, (d) specific training in clinical neuropsychology. This should include an 1800-hour internship which should be preceded by appropriate practicum experience.

(A) GENERIC PSYCHOLOGY CORE

1. Statistics and Methodology

2. Learning, Cognition, and Perception

3. Social Psychology and Personality

4. Physiological Psychology

5. Life-Span Developmental

6. History

(B) GENERIC CLINICAL CORE

1. Psychopathology

2. Psychometric Theory

3. Interview and Assessment Techniques

    i. Interviewing

    ii. Intelligence Assessment

    iii. Personality Assessment

4. Intervention Techniques

    i. Counseling and Psychotherapy

    ii. Behavior Therapy/Modification

    iii. Consultation

5. Professional Ethics

(C) NEUROSCIENCES AND BASIC HUMAN AND ANIMAL
    NEUROPSYCHOLOGY

  i. Basic Neurosciences

  ii. Advanced Physiological Psychology and Pharmacology

  iii. Neuropsychology of Perceptual, Cognitive, and Executive Processes

  iv. Research Design and Research Practicum in Neuropsychology

(D) SPECIFIC CLINICAL NEUROPSYCHOLOGICAL TRAINING

  i. Clinical Neurology and Neuropathology

  ii. Specialized neuropsychological assessment techniques

  iii. Specialized neuropsychological intervention techniques

  iv. Assessment practicum (children and/or adults) in University-supervised assessment
     facility

  v. Intervention practicum in University supervised intervention facility

  vi. Clinical Neuropsychological Internship of 1800 hours preferably in noncaptive facility.
     (As per INS/Div. 40 Task Force guidelines). Ordinarily this internship will be
     completed in a single year, but in exceptional circumstance may be completed in a
     2-year period.

(E) DOCTORAL DISSERTATION

It is recognized that the completion of a Ph.D. in Clinical Neuropsychology prepares the
person to begin work as a clinical neuropsychologist. In most jurisdictions, an additional
year of supervised clinical practice will be required in order to qualify for licensure.

Furthermore, training at the postdoctoral level to increase both general and subspecialty competencies is viewed as desirable.

Guidelines for Neuropsychology Internships in Clinical Neuropsychology

The following report summarizes the recommendations of the subcommittee on internships of the INS/Division 40 Task Force. The report was prepared by Linus Bieliauskas and Thomas Boll.

At the outset, it is recognized that the Internship Program is designed primarily for students with degrees in clinical psychology. Such internship programs are those accredited by the American Psychological Association and or those listed in the Directory of the Association of Psychology Internship Centers.

Entry into a psychology internship program is a minimum qualification in a Neuropsychology Internship. Such entry must be based on completion of at least 2 years in a recognized Psychology Ph.D. Graduate Training Program in an area of Health Services Delivery (e.g., Clinical, Clinical Neuropsychology, Counseling, or School Psychology). Alternately, entry into a psychology internship program must be based on completion of a "retreading" Program designed to meet equivalent criteria as a Health Services Delivery Program per se. Within the training programs described above, the student must also have completed a designated track, specialization, or concentration in neuropsychology

There are generally two models for psychology internship training: (I) Generic Clinical Psychology, and (2) specialty in Clinical Neuropsychology. The former does not concern us here since such training is not geared toward producing specialized experience or qualification. The latter type of internship program, when designed to provide specialized training in Neuropsychology, is what constitutes a Clinical Neuropsychology Internship.

A Clinical Neuropsychology Internship must devote at least 50% of a 1-year full-time training experience to neuropsychology. In addition, at least 20% of the training experience must be devoted to General Clinical Training to assure a competent background in Clinical Psychology. Such an internship should be associated with a hospital setting which has Neurological and/or Neurosurgical services to offer to the training background. Such an internship should not be associated only with a strictly psychiatric setting.

EXPERIENCES TO BE PROVIDED

The experiences to be provided to the intern in clinical neuropsychology should conform to the descriptions of professional activities in the Report of the Task Force on Education, Accreditation, and Credentialing of the International Neuropsychological Society and the American Psychological Associaton (198 1). Necessary training should be provided in both a didactic and experiential format. Supervisors in such an internship should be board-certified clinical neuropsychologists.

DIDACTIC TRAINING

A. Training in neurological diagnosis.

B. Training in consultation to neurological and neurosurgical services.

C. Training in direct consultation to psychiatric, pediatric, or general medical services.

D. Exposure to methods and practices of neurological and neurosurgical consultation (grand rounds, bed rounds, seminars, etc).

E. Training in neuropsychological techniques, examination, interpretation of test results, report writing.

F. Training in consultation to patients and referral sources.

G. Training in methods of intervention specific to clinical neuropsychology.

EXPERIENTIAL TRAINING

A. Neuropsychological examination and evaluation of patients with actual and suspected neurological diseases and disorders.

B. Neuropsychological examination and evaluation of patients with psychiatric disorders and/or pediatric or general medical patients with neurobehavioral disorders.

C. Participation in clinical activities with neurologists and neurosurgeons (bed rounds, grand rounds, etc.).

D. Direct consultation to patients involving neuropsychological issues.

E. Consultation to referral and treating professions.

EXIT CRITERIA

At the end of the internship year, the intern in clinical neuropsychology should be able to undertake consultation to patients and professionals on an independent basis and meet minimal qualifications for competent practice of clinical neuropsychology as defined in Section B, Neuropsychological roles and functions of the Report of the Task Force (1981).

Guidelines for Postdoctoral Training in Clinical Neuropsychology

Postdoctoral training, as described herein, is designed to provide clinical training to produce an advanced level of competence in the specialty of clinical neuropsychology. It is recognized that clinical neuropsychology is a scientifically based and evolving discipline and that such training should also provide a significant research component. Thus, this report is concerned with postdoctoral training in clinical neuropsychology which is specifically geared toward producing independent practioner level competence which includes both necessary clinical and research skills. This report does not address training in neuropsychology which is focused solely on research.

ENTRY CRITERIA

Entry into a clinical neuropsychology postdoctoral training program ordinarily should be based on completion of a regionally accredited Ph.D. graduate training program in one of the health service delivery areas of psychology or a Ph.D. in psychology with additional completion of a "respecialization" program designed to meet equivalent criteria as a health services delivery program in psychology. In all cases, candidacy for postdoctoral training in clinical neuropsychology must be based on demonstration of training and research methodology designed to meet equivalent criteria as a health services delivery professional in the scientist-practitioner model. Ordinarily, a clinical internship, listed by the Association of Psychology Internship Centers, must also have been completed.

GENERAL CONSIDERATIONS

A postdoctoral training program in clinical neuropsychology should be directed by a board-certified clinical neuropsychologist. In most cases, the program should extend over at least a 2-year period. The only exception would be for individuals who have completed a specific clinical neuropsychology specialization in their graduate programs and/or a clinical neuropsychology internship (Subcommittee Report of the Task Force, 1984) provided the exit criteria are met (see below). As a general guideline, the postdoctoral training program should provide at least 50% time in clinical service and at least 25% time in clinical research. Variance within these guidelines should be tailored to the needs of the individual. Specific training in neuropsychology must be provided, including any areas where the individual is deemed to be deficient (testing, consultation, intervention, neurosciences, neurology, etc.).

SPECIFIC CONSIDERATIONS

Such a postdoctoral training program should be associated with hospital settings which have neurological and/or neurosurgical services to offer to the training background. Necessary training should be provided in both a didactic and experiential format and should include the following:

DIDACTIC TRAINING

A. Training in neurological and psychiatric diagnosis.

B. Training in consultation to neurological and neurosurgical services.

C. Training in direct consultation to psychiatric, pediatric, or general medical services.

D. Exposure to methods and practices of neurological and neurosurgical consultation (Grand Rounds, Bed Rounds, Seminars, etc.).

E. Observation of neurosurgical procedures and biomedical tests (Revascularization procedures, cerebral blood flow, Wada testing, etc.).

F. Participation in seminars offered to neurology and neurosurgery residents (Neuropharmacology, EEG, brain-cutting, etc.).

G. Training in neuropsychological techniques, examination, interpretation of test results, report writing.

H. Training in consultation to patients and referral sources.

I. Training in methods of intervention specific to clinical neuropsychology.

J. Seminars, readings, etc., in neuropsychology (case conferences, journal discussion, topic-specific seminars).

K. Didactic training in neuroanatomy, neuropathology, and related neurosciences.

EXPERIENTIAL TRAINING

A. Neuropsychological examination and evaluation of patients with actual and suspected neurological diseases and disorders.

B. Neuropsychological examination and evaluation of patients with psychiatric disorders and/or pediatric or general medical patients with neurobehavioral disorders.

C. Participation in clinical activities with neurologists and neurosurgeons (bed rounds, grand rounds, etc.).

D. Experience at a specialty clinic, such as a dementia clinic or epilepsy clinic, which emphasizes multidisciplinary approaches to diagnosis and treatment.

E. Direct consultation to patients involving neuropsychological assessment.

F. Direct intervention with patients, specific to neuropsychological issues, and to include psychotherapy and/or family therapy where indicated.

G. Research in neuropsychology, i.e., collaboration on a research project or other scholarly academic activity, initiation of an independent research project or other scholarly academic activity, and presentation or publication of research data where appropriate.

EXIT CRITERIA

At the conclusion of the postdoctoral training program, the individual should be able to undertake consultation to patients and professionals on an independent basis. Accomplishment in research should also be demonstrated. The program is designed to produce a competent practitioner in the areas designated in Section B of the Task Force Report (1981) and to provide eligibility for external credentialing and licensure as designated in section D of the Task Force Report (1981). The latter also includes training eligibility for certification in Clinical Neuropsychology by the American Board of Professional Psychology.

References

Meier, M.J. (1981). Report of the Task Force on Education, Accreditation and Credentialing of the International Neuropsychological Society. *The INS Bulletin,* September, pp. 5–10.

Report of the Task Force on Education, Accreditation, and Credentialing. *The INS Bulletin,* 1981, pp. 5–10. *Newsletter 40,* 1984, 2, 3–8.

Report of the Subcommittee on Psychology Internships. *Newsletter 40,* 1984, *2, 7. The INS Bulletin,* 1984, p. 33, *APIC Newsletter,* 1983, 9, 27–28.

APPENDIX B

Division 40 (1989): Definition of a Clinical Neuropsychologist

Text reprinted with permission from Taylor & Francis.

Division 40, (1989). Definition of a clinical neuropsychologist. *The Clinical Neuropsychologist*, 3, 22.

Professional Issues

Definition of a Clinical Neuropsychologist

The Following Statement was Adopted by the Executive Committee Of Division 40 At The Apa Meeting On August 12, 1988

A Clinical Neuropsychologist is a professional psychologist who applies principles of assessment and intervention based upon the scientific study of human behavior as it relates to normal and abnormal functioning of the central nervous system. The Clinical Neuropsychologist is a doctoral-level psychology provider of diagnostic and intervention services who has demonstrated competence in the application of such principles for human welfare following:

A. Successful completion of systematic didactic and experiential training in neuropsychology and neuroscience at a regionally accredited university;

B. Two or more years of appropriate supervised training applying neuropsychological services in a clinical setting;

C. Licensing and certification to provide psychological services to the public by the laws of the state or province in which he or she practices:

D. Review by one's peers as a test of these competencies. Attainment of the ABCNIABPP Diploma in Clinical Neuropsychology is the clearest evidence of competence as a Clinical Neuropsychologist, assuring that all of these criteria have been met.

Attainment of the ABCNIABPP Diploma in Clinical Neuropsychology is the clearest evidence of competence as a Clinical Neuropsychologist, assuring that all of these criteria have been met.

This statement reflects the official position of the Division of Clinical Neuropsychology and should not be construed as either contrary to or supraordinate to the policies of the APA at large.

Public Description of Clinical Neuropsychology 2010

Clinical Neuropsychology is a specialty in professional psychology that applies principles of assessment and intervention based upon the scientific study of human behavior as it relates to normal and abnormal functioning of the central nervous system. The specialty is dedicated to enhancing the understanding of brain-behavior relationships and the application of such knowledge to human problems.

Specialized Knowledge

Specialized knowledge and training in the applied science of brain-behavior relationships is foundational to the specialty of clinical neuropsychology. In addition to foundational and functional competencies in professional psychology, clinical neuropsychologists have specialized knowledge of functional neuroanatomy, principles of neuroscience, brain development, neurological disorders and etiologies, neurodiagnostic techniques, normal and abnormal brain functioning, and neuropsychological and behavioral manifestations of neurological disorders. Preparation in clinical neuropsychology begins at the doctoral level and specialized education and training is completed at the postdoctoral level.

Problems Addressed

Clinical neuropsychologists address neurobehavioral problems related to acquired or developmental disorders of the nervous system. The types of problems are extremely varied and include such conditions as dementia, vascular disorders, Parkinson's disease and other neurodegenerative disorders, traumatic brain injury, seizure disorders, learning disabilities, neuropsychiatric disorders, infectious disease affecting the CNS, neurodevelopmental disorders, metabolic disease, and neurological effects of medical disorders or treatment.

Populations Served

Clinical neuropsychologists apply specialized knowledge in the assessment, diagnosis, treatment, and rehabilitation of individuals with neurological, medical, or neurodevelopmental disorders across the lifespan. Pediatric neuropsychologists provide clinical services to children and adolescents (and their families).

Skills and Procedures Utilized

Clinical neuropsychologists are skilled in clinical assessment and treatment of brain disorders. Essential skills include specialized neuropsychological assessment techniques, specialized intervention techniques, research design and analysis in neuropsychology, professional issues and ethics, culturally competent approaches in neuropsychology, and understanding of implications of neuropsychological conditions for behavior and adjustment. Competence in clinical neuropsychology requires the ability to integrate neuropsychological findings with neurologic and other medical data, psychosocial and other behavioral data, and knowledge in the neurosciences, and interpret these findings with an appreciation of social, cultural and ethical issues.

The Houston Conference on Specialty Education and Training in Clinical Neuropsychology Policy Statement

Text reprinted with permission from the National Academy of Neuropsychology.

The Houston Conference on Specialty Education and Training in Clinical Neuropsychology

Policy Statement

I. PREAMBLE FOR CONFERENCE.

Clinical neuropsychology is a specialty formally recognized by the American Psychological Association (APA) and the Canadian Psychological Association (CPA). Education and training in clinical neuropsychology has evolved along with the development of the specialty itself. Nevertheless, there has been no widely recognized and accepted description of integrated education and training in the specialty of clinical neuropsychology The aim of the Houston Conference was to advance an aspirational, integrated model of specialty training in clinical neuropsychology.

The Conference Planning Committee solicited participant applications by way of an announcement in the APA Monitor and letters to members of the Division of Clinical Neuropsychology (Division 40), the National Academy of Neuropsychology (NAN), and to the directors of training programs at the doctoral, internship, and postdoctoral levels as listed in The Clinical Neuropsychologist (Cripe, 1995). The committee selected a group of 37 clinical neuropsychologists to reflect diversity in practice settings, education and training models, specializations in the field of clinical neuropsychology, levels of seniority, culture, geographic location, and sex. Five additional delegates attended as representatives of the sponsoring neuropsychological organizations (NAN; Division 40; the American Board of Clinical Neuropsychology [ABCN]; the American Academy of Clinical Neuropsychology [AACN]; and the Association of Postdoctoral Programs in Clinical Neuropsychology [APPCN]). These delegates convened in Houston from September 3 through September 7, 1997. This document is the product of their deliberations. [Additional details may be found in the Proceedings of the Houston Conference.]

II. INTRODUCTION.

The following document is a description of integrated education and training in the specialty of clinical neuropsychology. It is predicated on the view that the training of the specialist in clinical neuropsychology must be scientist-practitioner based, and may lead to a combined, primarily practice, or primarily academic career.

The scientist-practitioner model (Belar & Perry, 1992) as applied to clinical neuropsychology envisions that all aspects of general neuropsychology and professional education and training should be integrated; this is the "horizontal" dimension of education and training. Integration should begin with doctoral education and should continue through internship and residency education and training; this is the "vertical" dimension of education and training.

This document presents a model of integrated education and training in the specialty of clinical neuropsychology that is both programmatic and competency-based (see Section XV below). This model defines exit criteria and provides tracks and means for obtaining these criteria across all levels of education and training. Exit criteria for the completion of specialty training are met by the end of the residency program. The programmatic level at which these criteria are achieved may vary but not the content.

III. WHO IS A CLINICAL NEUROPSYCHOLOGIST?

A clinical neuropsychologist is a professional psychologist trained in the science of brain-behavior relationships. The clinical neuropsychologist specializes in the application of assessment and intervention principles based on the scientific study of human behavior across the lifespan as it relates to normal and abnormal functioning of the central nervous system.

IV. WHO SHOULD HAVE EDUCATION AND TRAINING IN THE SPECIALTY OF CLINICAL NEUROPSYCHOLOGY?

1. Persons who engage in the specialty practice of clinical neuropsychology or supervise the specialty practice of clinical neuropsychology.
2. Persons who call themselves "clinical neuropsychologists" or otherwise designate themselves as engaging in the specialty practice of clinical neuropsychology.
3. Psychologists who engage in educating or supervising trainees in the specialty practice of clinical neuropsychology.

V. PROFESSIONAL AND SCIENTIFIC ACTIVITY.

The clinical neuropsychologist's professional activities are included within the seven core domains delineated in the Petition for the Recognition of a Specialty in Professional Psychology submitted by Division 40 of the APA to the Commission for the Recognition of Specialties and Proficiencies in Professional Psychology (CRSPPP). These core domains are: assessment, intervention, consultation, supervision, research and inquiry, consumer protection, and professional development. The scientific activities of the specialist in clinical neuropsychology can vary widely. The specialist whose professional activities involve diverse cultural, ethnic, and linguistic populations has the knowledge and skills to perform those activities competently and ethically. The essential knowledge and skill competencies for these activities are outlined below.

VI. KNOWLEDGE BASE.

Clinical neuropsychologists possess the following knowledge. This core knowledge may be acquired through multiple pathways, not limited to courses, and may come through other documentable didactic methods.

1. Generic Psychology Core

    A. Statistics and methodology

    B. Learning, cognition and perception

    C. Social psychology and personality

    D. Biological basis of behavior

    E. Life span development

    F. History

    G. Cultural and individual differences and diversity

2. Generic Clinical Core

    A. Psychopathology

    B. Psychometric theory

    C. Interview and assessment techniques

    D. Intervention techniques

    E. Professional ethics

3. Foundations for the study of brain-behavior relationships

    A. Functional neuroanatomy

    B. Neurological and related disorders including their etiology, pathology, course and treatment

    C. Non-neurologic conditions affecting CNS functioning

    D. Neuroimaging and other neurodiagnostic techniques

    E. Neurochemistry of behavior (e.g., psychopharmacology)

    F. Neuropsychology of behavior

4. Foundations for the practice of clinical neuropsychology

    A. Specialized neuropsychological assessment techniques

    B. Specialized neuropsychological intervention techniques

    C. Research design and analysis in neuropsychology

    D. Professional issues and ethics in neuropsychology

    E. Practical implications of neuropsychological conditions

VII. SKILLS.

Clinical neuropsychologists possess the following generic clinical skills and skills in clinical neuropsychology. These core skills may be acquired through multiple pathways, not limited to courses, and may come through other documentable didactic methods. Domains of skills and examples are:

1. Assessment

    • Information gathering

    • History taking

- Selection of tests and measures
- Administration of tests and measures
- Interpretation and diagnosis
- Treatment planning
- Report writing
- Provision of feedback
- Recognition of multicultural issues

2. Treatment and Interventions

- Identification of intervention targets
- Specification of intervention needs
- Formulation of an intervention plan
- Implementation of the plan
- Monitoring and adjustment to the plan as needed
- Assessment of the outcome
- Recognition of multicultural issues

3. Consultation (patients, families, medical colleagues, agencies, etc.)

- Effective basic communication (e.g., listening, explaining, negotiating)
- Determination and clarification of referral issues
- Education of referral sources regarding neuropsychological services (strengths and limitations)
- Communication of evaluation results and recommendations
- Education of patients and families regarding services and disorder(s)

4. Research

- Selection of appropriate research topics
- Review of relevant literature
- Design of research
- Execution of research
- Monitoring of progress
- Evaluation of outcome
- Communication of results

5. Teaching and Supervision

- Methods of effective teaching
- Plan and design of courses and curriculums
- Use of effective educational technologies

- Use of effective supervision methodologies (assessment, intervention, and research)
- It is recognized that the relative weightings of these dimensions may vary from one program to another.

VIII. DOCTORAL EDUCATION IN CLINICAL NEUROPSYCHOLOGY.

Specialization in clinical neuropsychology begins at the doctoral level which provides the generic psychology and clinical core. In addition, it includes foundations for the study of brain-behavior relations and the practice of clinical neuropsychology. All of these are specified above in Sections VI and VII.

Doctoral education in clinical neuropsychology occurs at a regionally accredited institution. All basic aspects of the generic psychology and generic clinical cores should be completed at the doctoral level. The foundation of brain-behavior relationships should be developed to a considerable degree at this level of training. Yet, variability may occur between doctoral programs in the degree to which foundations of brain-behavior relationships and clinical neuropsychology practice are emphasized.

Entry and exit criteria for this level are those specified by the doctoral program.

IX. INTERNSHIP TRAINING IN CLINICAL NEUROPSYCHOLOGY.

The purpose of the internship is to complete training in the general practice of professional psychology and extend specialty preparation in science and professional practice in clinical neuropsychology. The percentage of time in clinical neuropsychology should be determined by the training needs of the individual intern.

Internships must be completed in an APA or CPA approved professional psychology training program. Internship entry requirements are the completion of all graduate education and training requirements including the completion of the doctoral dissertation.

X. RESIDENCY EDUCATION AND TRAINING IN CLINICAL NEUROPSYCHOLOGY.

Residency education and training is designed to provide clinical, didactic and academic training to produce an advanced level of competence in the specialty of clinical neuropsychology and to complete the education and training necessary for independent practice in the specialty. The postdoctoral residency program is a required component in specialty education in clinical neuropsychology. The expected period of residency extends for the equivalent of two years of full-time education and training. The residency experience must occur on at least a half-time basis.

These programs will pursue accreditation supporting the following assurances.

1. The faculty is comprised of a board-certified clinical neuropsychologist and other professional psychologists;

2. Training is provided at a fixed site or on formally affiliated and geographically proximate training sites, with primarily on-site supervision;

3. There is access to clinical services and training programs in medical specialties and allied professions;

4. There are interactions with other residents in medical specialties and allied professions, if not other residents in clinical neuropsychology;

5. Each resident spends significant percentages of time in clinical service, and clinical research, and educational activities, appropriate to the individual resident's training needs.

Entry into a clinical neuropsychology residency program should be based upon completion of an APA or CPA accredited doctoral education and training program. Clinical neuropsychology residents will have successfully completed an APA or CPA accredited internship program which includes some training in clinical neuropsychology.

Exit criteria for the residency are as follows:

1. Advanced skill in the neuropsychological evaluation, treatment and consultation to patients and professionals sufficient to practice on an independent basis;

2. Advanced understanding of brain-behavior relationships;

3. Scholarly activity, e.g., submission of a study or literature review for publication, presentation, submission of a grant proposal or outcome assessment.

4. A formal evaluation of competency in the exit criteria 1 through 3 shall occur in the residency program.

5. Eligibility for state or provincial licensure or certification for the independent practice of psychology.

6. Eligibility for board certification in clinical neuropsychology by the American Board of Professional Psychology.

XI. NATURE AND PLACE OF SUBSPECIALTIES WITHIN CLINICAL NEUROPSYCHOLOGY.

In the future, subspecialties in clinical neuropsychology may be recognized (e.g., child, pediatric, geriatric, rehabilitation). In fact, many clinical neuropsychologists currently concentrate their professional and scientific activities in relatively focused areas of the clinical neuropsychology specialty. Thus, it is expected that some or all of these areas of concentration will eventually be seen as bona fide subspecialties. One implication of this view is that residencies may emerge that reflect concentrations in these subspecialties.

XII. CONTINUING EDUCATION IN CLINICAL NEUROPSYCHOLOGY.

All specialists in clinical neuropsychology are expected to engage in annual continuing education. The goal of continuing education is to enhance or maintain the already established competence of clinical neuropsychologists by updating previously acquired knowledge and skills or by acquiring new knowledge or skills. Continuing education is not a method for acquiring core knowledge or skills to practice clinical neuropsychology or identify oneself as a clinical neuropsychologist. Continuing education also should not be the primary vehicle for career changes from another specialty area in psychology to clinical neuropsychology.

XIII. DIVERSITY IN EDUCATION AND TRAINING.

The specialty of clinical neuropsychology should attempt to actively involve (enroll, recruit) individuals from diverse backgrounds at all levels of education and training in clinical neuropsychology.

XIV. APPLICATION OF THE MODEL.

This document is not to be applied retroactively to individuals currently trained or in training in the specialty of clinical neuropsychology. Individuals entering the specialty or training for the specialty of clinical neuropsychology prior to the implementation of this document are governed by existing standards as to the appropriateness of identifying themselves as clinical neuropsychologists.

XV. MODEL OF INTEGRATED EDUCATION AND TRAINING IN CLINICAL NEUROPSYCHOLOGY.

Figure 1 demonstrates how different degrees of specialty knowledge and skills (horizontal dimension) are acquired at various levels of training (vertical dimension). The model facilitates longitudinal integration and continuity in knowledge and skill acquisition with an emphasis that will vary according to level of training. The two charts show the education and training sequence for (A) an individual who acquires some of these areas primarily at

FIGURE A1:

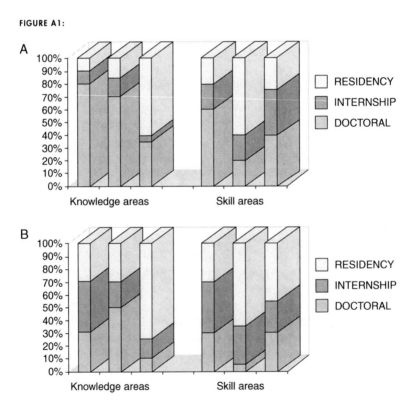

the doctoral level and (B) an individual who acquires some of these areas to a lesser degree at the doctoral level and much greater degree at the internship and residency levels.

An illustration of an integrated model of education and training in clinical neuropsychology.

From: Hannay, H. J., Bieliauskas, L. A., Crosson, B. A., Hammeke, T. A., Hamsher, K. deS., & Koffler, S. P. (1998). Proceedings: The Houston Conference on Specialty Education and Training in Clinical Neuropsychology. *Archives of Clinical Neuropsychology*, *13*(2). Copyright by the National Academy of Neuropsychology. Reproduced with permission.

References

Cripe, L. L. (1995). Special Division 40 presentation: Listing of Training Programs in Clinical Neuropsychology - 1995. *The Clinical Neuropsychologist*, *9*, 327–398.

Belar, C. D., & Perry, N. W. (1992). National Conference on Scientist-Practitioner Education and Training for the Professional Practice of Psychology. *American Psychologist*, *47*, 71–75. Downloaded January 11, 2011 from http://www.theaacn.org/position_papers/Houston_Conference.pdf.

National Academy of Neuropsychology Approved Definition of a Clinical Neuropsychologist

Text reprinted with permission from the National Academy of Neuropsychology.

Nan Definition of a Clinical Neuropsychologist 2001

Official Position of the National Academy of Neuropsychology
Approved by the Board of Directors 05/05/2001
This 2001 definition expands upon and modifies the 1989 definition by Division 40 of the American Psychological Association, which was used as the foundation for this updated document

A clinical neuropsychologist is a professional within the field of psychology with special expertise in the applied science of brain-behavior relationships. Clinical neuropsychologists use this knowledge in the assessment, diagnosis, treatment, and/or rehabilitation of patients across the lifespan with neurological, medical, neurodevelopmental and psychiatric conditions, as well as other cognitive and learning disorders. The clinical neuropsychologist uses psychological, neurological, cognitive, behavioral, and physiological principles, techniques and tests to evaluate patients' neurocognitive, behavioral, and emotional strengths and weaknesses and their relationship to normal and abnormal central nervous system functioning. The clinical neuropsychologist uses this information and information provided by other medical/health care providers to identify and diagnose neurobehavioral disorders, and plan and implement intervention strategies. The specialty of clinical neuropsychology is recognized by the American Psychological Association and the Canadian Psychological Association. Clinical neuropsychologists are independent practitioners (health care providers) of clinical neuropsychology and psychology.

The clinical neuropsychologist (minimal criteria) has:

1. A doctoral degree in psychology from an accredited university training program.

2. An internship, or its equivalent, in a clinically relevant area of professional psychology.

3. The equivalent of two (full-time) years of experience and specialized training, at least one of which is at the postdoctoral level, in the study and practice of clinical neuropsychology and related neurosciences. These two years include supervision by a clinical neuropsychologist[1].

---

[1] Individuals receiving training in clinical neuropsychology prior to this 2001 definition should be subject to the educational and experiential guidelines published by Division 40 of the American

4. A license in his or her state or province to practice psychology and/or clinical neuro-psychology independently, or is employed as a neuropsychologist by an exempt agency.

At present, board certification is not required for practice in clinical neuropsychology. Board certification (through formal credential verification, written and oral examination, and peer review) in the specialty of clinical neuropsychology is further evidence of the above advanced training, supervision, and applied fund of knowledge in clinical neuro-psychology.

References

Report of the Division 40/INS Joint Task Force on Education, Accreditation, and Credentialing (1984). *Division 40 Newsletter*, Vol.2, no. 2, pp. 3–8.

Definition of a Clinical Neuropsychologist, *The Clinical Neuropsychologist* 1989, Vol. 3, No. 1, pp.22

Psychological Association (APA, 1984; 1989). The 2001 definition should not be interpreted as negating the credentials of individuals whose education and experience predates the Division 40-apa defini-tions. Individuals meeting these prior criteria are and continue to be clinical neuropsychologists under this 2001 definition.

American Academy of Clinical Neuropsychology (AACN) Practice Guidelines for Neuropsychological Assessment and Consultation

Text reprinted with permission from Taylor & Francis and the American Academy of Clinical Neuropsychology.

American Academy of Clinical Neuropsychology (Aacn) Practice Guidelines for Neuropsychological Assessment and Consultation

BOARD OF DIRECTORS

American Academy of Clinical Neuropsychology

This document is the first set of practice guidelines to be formally reviewed and endorsed by the AACN Board of Directors and published in the official journal of AACN. They have been formulated with the assumption that guidelines and standards for neuropsychological assessment and consultation are essential to professional development. As such, they are intended to facilitate the continued systematic growth of the profession of clinical neuropsychology, and to help assure a high level of professional practice. These guidelines are offered to serve members of AACN, as well as the field of clinical neuropsychology as a whole.

Introduction

Clinical neuropsychology has experienced tremendous growth in recent years, whether measured in terms of the number of practitioners, scientific studies, meetings, journals, training programs, or assessment tools. Organizations devoted to neuropsychology have formed and have become well established, yet are still maturing. Within the American Psychological Association (APA), the Division of Clinical Neuropsychology (Division 40) was formed in 1980 and clinical neuropsychology was recognized as a specialty in 1996. Definitions of "neuropsychology" and core training requirements have been developed (Hannay et al., 1998) and a number of general approaches to performing valid and appropriate neuropsychological assessment are recognized as having common core features (cf. Lezak, Howieson, & Loring, 2004).

Identification of professional issues and explication of standards is essential to providing quality neuropsychological services to the public and to developing neuropsychology as a science and clinical specialty. Development of guidelines for neuropsychological assessment is the next logical step in the growth, development, and maturation of the field of clinical neuropsychology. In the era of evidence-based practice in psychology (EBPP), such guidelines should be "based on careful systematic weighing of research data and clinical expertise" (APA, 2006). The present document is founded on the assumptions that standards for neuropsychological assessment and consultation are essential to professional development and protection of the public, and that such standards can be articulated as general aspirational guidelines despite theoretical and practical diversity within the field (APA, 2005). Consistent with its mission, the American Academy of Clinical Neuropsychology (AACN) is in a position to take on this responsibility. The present Guidelines are offered to serve members of AACN, as well as the profession of neuro-psychology as a whole.

The American Board of Clinical Neuropsychology (ABCN) is a member specialty examining board under a unitary governing body, the American Board of Professional Psychology (ABPP). Founded in 1947, ABPP is the oldest peer-reviewed board for psychol-ogy and grants board certification in several specialty areas of psychology, including clinical neuropsychology. Within ABPP, ABCN is responsible for the examination process for clinical neuropsychology board certification candidates, with AACN being the mem-bership organization for individuals who have been awarded board certification by ABCN. Inherent in this examination process are de facto and consensually accepted standards for training, knowledge, and clinical practice in neuropsychology (updated policy and proce-dures are available online at http://www.theabcn.org).

This document is intended to serve as a guide for the practice of neuropsychological assessment and consultation and is designed to promote quality and consistency in neuro-psychological evaluations. Psychologists may use these Guidelines to evaluate their own readiness to perform neuropsychological evaluations and as a framework for performing this type of work. Psychologists who desire to upgrade skills, knowledge, and experience may also use these Guidelines as a reference. Other organizations, disciplines, professionals, entities, and individuals are encouraged to consider these Guidelines as principles for the provision of neuropsychological services. Because they apply to the current practice of clinical neuropsychology, these Guidelines will require periodic review and are intended to remain in effect until a point in time at which the AACN Board of Directors (BOD) determines that a revision is necessary.

The present Guidelines are intended to be compatible with the current APA (2002b) Ethical Principles of Psychologists and Code of Conduct (EPPCC) and follow the recom-mendations of other APA documents, including the Criteria for Practice Guideline Development and Evaluation (2002a) and Determination and Documentation of the Need for Practice Guidelines (2005). The EPPCC are intended to describe standards for compe-tent and adequate professional conduct. In contrast to applicable codes of ethics, the pres-ent Guidelines are intended to describe the most desirable and highest level professional conduct for neuropsychologists when engaged in the practice of clinical neuropsychology. In the event of a conflict, the EPPCC or other AACN policy statements can inform the prac-tical use of these Guidelines. Similarly, applicable federal and state laws supersede these guidelines.

The term "guidelines" refers to statements that suggest or recommend specific profes-sional behavior, endeavors, or conduct for psychologists. The primary purpose of practice guidelines is to promote high-quality psychological services by providing the practitioner with well-supported practical guidance and education in a particular practice area. Practice guidelines also "inform psychologists, the public, and other interested parties regarding desirable professional conduct" (APA, 2005). Guidelines differ from "standards" in that standards are mandatory and may be accompanied by an enforcement mechanism, whereas guidelines are aspirational in intent. Guidelines are intended to facilitate the continued systematic development of the profession and to help assure a high level of professional practice (APA, 2005). They are not intended to be mandatory or exhaustive, and may not be applicable to every professional and clinical situation. They are not to be promulgated as a means of establishing the identity of a group or specialty area of psychology. Likewise, they are not created with the purpose of excluding any psychologist from practicing in a particular area, nor are they intended to take precedence over a psychologist's judgment.

Outline of the Guidelines

1. Definitions

2. Purpose and Scope

3. Education and Training

4. Work Settings

5. Ethical and Clinical Issues

    A. Informed consent

    B. Patient issues in third-party assessments

    C. Test security

    D. Underserved populations=cultural issues

6. Methods and Procedures

    A. The decision to evaluate

    B. Review of records

    C. Interview of patient and significant others

    D. Measurement procedures

    E. Assessment of motivation and effort

    F. Assessment of concurrent validity

    G. Test administration and scoring

    H. Interpretation

    I. The evaluation report

    J. Providing feedback

1. Definitions

Clinical neuropsychology has been defined as "an applied science concerned with the behavioral expression of brain function and dysfunction" (Lezak et al., 2004). Vanderploeg (2000) noted that neuropsychology studies "the impact of brain injury or disease on the cognitive, sensorimotor, emotional, and general adaptive capacities of the individual." In a similar vein, Prigatano (2002) offered that neuropsychology is "the scientific study of how the brain produces mind and how disorders of the brain cause a variety of mental and personality disturbances." Integrating these statements, *clinical neuropsychology is an applied science that examines the impact of both normal and abnormal brain functioning on a broad range of cognitive, emotional, and behavioral functions.* The distinctive features of neuropsychological evaluations and consultations in assessing brain function and dysfunction include the use of objective neuropsychological tests, systematic behavioral observations, and interpretation of the findings based on knowledge of the neuropsychological manifestations of brain-related conditions. Where appropriate, these evaluations consider neuroimaging and other neurodiagnostic studies and inform neuropsychologically oriented rehabilitation interventions.

2. Purpose and Scope

Clinical neuropsychologists conduct their professional activities in accord with the EPPCC (APA, 2002b), and any AACN position statements that apply to particular issues or areas of practice that are relevant to their professional activities. They are also aware of and may seek guidance from the standards of practice and principles of other relevant professional organizations (e.g., American Academy of Forensic Psychology, American Academy of Pediatrics).

While the professional standards for the ethical practice of psychology are addressed in the EPPCC, these principles are not fully inclusive with respect to the current aspirations of desirable professional conduct for clinical neuropsychologists. By design, none of the present Guidelines contradicts any of the principles of the EPPCC; rather, they exemplify those principles in the context of the practice of clinical neuropsychology, as herein defined. The Guidelines have been designed to be national in scope and are intended to conform to applicable state and federal law. In situations in which the clinical neuropsychologist believes that the requirements of law are in conflict with these Guidelines, attempts to resolve the conflict should be made in accordance with the procedures set forth in the EPPCC.

The present Guidelines specify the nature of desirable professional practice by clinical neuropsychologists within any subdiscipline of this specialty (e.g., child, forensic). The term "psychologist" designates any individual whose professional activities are defined by APA and by regulation of title by state registration or licensure, as the practice of psychology. "Clinical neuropsychologist" refers to psychologists who engage in the practice of clinical neuropsychology as defined above.

3. Education and Training

Early in the development of the field of clinical neuropsychology, neuropsychologists were in limited demand, and there were few formal training programs. By 1979, the International Neuropsychological Society (INS) had published broad guidelines indicating alternative pathways for obtaining competence in this discipline (Rourke & Murji, 2000). At one point, a formal re-specialization program of continuing education was suggested as one means of helping psychologists gain the necessary skills to practice neuropsychology. Continuing education, however, is only intended to expand or elaborate on established skills and is not regarded as an adequate modality for establishing competence in neuropsychology (Bornstein, 1988a). Formal training programs are now widely available (Cripe, 2000; Donders, 2002), and the nature of specialized neuropsychological training has been defined (Bornstein, 1988b; Hannay et al., 1998) and is the basis for the Guidelines proposed herein.

As evident from the definition of neuropsychology, a neuropsychologist possesses skills beyond simply administering and scoring a particular set of tests (Matarazzo, 1990; Meyer et al., 2001). A neuropsychologist is "a professional psychologist trained in the science of brain-behavior relationships" (Hannay et al., 1998). Kane, Goldstein, and Parsons (1989) pointed out that "the unique competence of the neuropsychologist is that of conceptualizing assessment results within a brain-behavior framework." The prefix "neuro" in neuropsychologist means that the psychologist is a specialist who has had explicit training in neuroscience and neurological bases of behavior. To fulfill this role, neuropsychologists must have specialized knowledge and training, a fact that is incorporated into the existing definitions of a neuropsychologist (Barth et al., 2003; Bieliauskas, 1999). Both APA Division 40 (Clinical Neuropsychology) and the National Academy of Neuropsychology (NAN) definitions require 2 years of specialized training. The APA Division 40 definition requires formal university training in neuropsychology and the neurosciences, and recommends a peer review process as an indicator of competency. The NAN definition (National Academy of Neuropsychology, 2001) requires, for individuals receiving training after 2001, "the equivalent of two (full-time) years of experience and specialized training, at least one of which is at the postdoctoral level, in the study and practice of clinical neuropsychology and related neurosciences. These two years include supervision by a clinical neuropsychologist."

4. Work Settings

Clinical neuropsychologists comprise a relatively small group compared with other specialists in the health care marketplace. Indeed, according to recent SAMHSA Mental Health Information Center statistics (http://www.mentalhealth.samhsa.gov/publications/allpubs/ SMA01–3537/chapter20.asp), there are over 77,000 licensed doctoral-level psychologists in the United States. At present, there are roughly 4,000 individuals purporting to practice clinical neuropsychology in the United States as reflected by membership in APA Division 40. This is a small number relative to other organizations including the 7,000 members of Division 12 (Clinical Psychology) of APA, 17,000 members of the American Academy of Neurology (AAN), and over 150,000 members of APA. Nonetheless, from the beginning of its development in the United States in the 1950s and 1960s, clinical neuropsychology has flourished as a discipline because of its unique focus and clinical utility.

The settings in which clinical neuropsychologists practice are richly varied. To illustrate, a neuropsychological text edited by Lamberty, Courtney, and Heilbronner (2003) includes chapters from practitioners who work in independent practice, collaborate with physicians in a medical practice, forensic settings (e.g., civil and correctional), or have adult and child practices in rural or urban communities, university affiliated medical centers, university-based attention deficit-hyperactivity disorder (ADHD) and learning disorder clinics, Veterans Affairs medical centers, general hospital settings, medical rehabilitation units, or schools. Other practice environments include military bases, pharmaceutical companies, surgical centers, and practices in which patients for social security and disability benefits are evaluated (Sweet, Peck, Abramowitz, & Etzweiler, 2000). Neuropsychologists have established themselves and the utility of neuropsychology as a specialty practice, in a number of medical, legal, social service, and other professional settings (Prigatano & Pliskin, 2003).

5. Ethical and Clinical Issues

The following section identifies four ethical and clinical issues that are particularly relevant to the practice of clinical neuropsychology and to the development of these guidelines. However, many other practice-related issues, such as effects of third-party observers and the use of psychometricians, are not covered. The reader is referred to relevant AACN position papers or documents from other membership organizations for discussion of these and other issues (see http://www.theaacn.org and http://www.nanonline.org).

A. INFORMED CONSENT

Neuropsychologists are aware of, and sensitive to, ethical and legal issues of informed consent, confidentiality, autonomy, and related human rights that arise in the context of evaluating children and adults. This is also true for "vulnerable adults," such as patients with mental retardation, developmental disabilities, or dementia, including those who already have designated legal guardians. The limits of confidentiality are explained to all examinees (or to parents or guardians, when appropriate) at the outset of a neuropsychological evaluation. The neuropsychologist establishes a clear understanding of examiner–examinee relationship issues, and ensures that this understanding is shared with the examinee and, if necessary, with relevant third parties, such as a referring physician, social worker, special education administrator, or attorney, and in some cases with insurers (Johnson-Greene & NAN Policy & Planning Committee, 2005). Consideration of such relationships is critical in identifying the person legally entitled to consent to the evaluation and to a release of information about the examinee. The following questions might be asked in these situations: For a patient with dementia or mental retardation, is there a court-appointed guardian? For a child, if the parents are divorced, who has legal custody to give consent for the evaluation and who has a right to receive full disclosure of the findings?

B. PATIENT ISSUES IN THIRD-PARTY ASSESSMENTS

Neuropsychologists may evaluate someone at the request of a third party (e.g., insurance carrier, attorney, judge, or special education hearing officer), as part of a legal proceeding, a disability evaluation, or special education due process hearings. In such cases, the neuropsychologist clarifies the nature of the relationship with the referring third party by establishing that the neuropsychologist will provide a candid and objective opinion based on the evaluation results (Bush & NAN Policy & Planning Committee, 2005a). In a legal dispute, such an opinion is offered regardless of whether the referral comes from someone advocating for the examinee or for a different party.

At the outset of the evaluation, the neuropsychologist establishes the aims of the assessment, describes in clear language the sorts of information requested of the patient and types of testing procedures to be performed, the general information- gathering procedures to be followed (e.g., whether the evaluation will involve formal standardized testing, interview, observation in the office, observations in natural settings such as school, home, or daycare, or collection of information from collateral sources where deemed appropriate, such as care providers, teachers, health aides, parents, spouse), the means of providing feedback (e.g., oral and=or written), and to whom and when a neuropsychological report will be sent. The neuropsychologist and referring parties discuss in advance who will pay for the evaluation, what costs are anticipated, and what payment arrangements can be made. In the case of a third-party referral, the neuropsychologist explains to the examinee (or guardians) that the party requesting the evaluation, rather than the patient being evaluated, is considered the "client," at least in the sense that it is this party that will receive the evaluation findings and report. The examinee is helped to understand that his=her responses, and the neuropsychologist's opinions about him=her, will be shared with the referring party, and that the referring party will decide how to use the information (e.g., whether it will be given to opposing attorneys, read aloud in court, etc.). The information from the examination may also be used in future or separate legal or administrative proceedings. The examinee is entitled to decline to participate, but the neuropsychologist should advise him=her to consult with his=her attorney or agent to clarify the possible consequences of consenting, or refusing, to be evaluated. Written reports, in these circumstances, clearly avoid the implication of patienthood or ongoing treatment and identify the examinee as distinct from the name and social=legal identity of the referral source.

In forensic cases, neuropsychologists are careful to distinguish between the role of an "expert" and the role of a "clinician." The expert's role is to inform the attorney(s), as well as the "trier of fact" (e.g., a judge, jury, or hearing officer) of the neuropsychological findings and to present unbiased opinions and answers to specific questions pertinent to the case, based on relevant scientific and clinical evidence (i.e., to be an "advocate of the facts") of the case. In contrast, the treating clinician's role is to be an advocate for his=her patient. Taking on the role of a patient advocate in a forensic situation might be perceived as biasing the clinician's opinions in favor of the patient. The neuropsychologist acting as a forensic expert typically does not conduct a feedback and treatment-planning conference with examinees (or their representative). A neuropsychologist who has treated a patient generally will decline to serve as an expert with regard to that case. If called upon to testify, the treating clinician responds in a manner consistent with original role limitations and qualifies his=her role when answering questions about the patient.

Neuropsychologists may provide a "second opinion" based on a review of another neuropsychologist's report, at the request of a judge or an attorney, an insurance company, or another psychologist. In this situation, the neuropsychologist is careful to base such an opinion only on available data and to express caution when lacking the information to provide a more substantive basis for their opinion(s). For example, the neuropsychologist may not be certain about the quality of examiner–examinee rapport or the accuracy of test administration procedures for the evaluation under review, or may find it difficult to form opinions based on the tests administered. Therefore, the "second opinion" might be limited to statements regarding whether or not the other examiner chose appropriate tests, reported the scores accurately, and made inferences, conclusions, and recommendations that are supported by the data provided in the report; whether alternative conclusions or recommendations, not mentioned in the report, should be considered; and whether any further neuropsychological tests or other information gathering (e.g., medical examinations) should be carried out to answer questions relevant to the case.

C. TEST SECURITY

Appropriate test security is the assumed responsibility of any practicing neuropsychologist and reflects several different levels for maintaining the safekeeping and utility of any test. Likewise, how the test results are disseminated to patients also falls under the guidelines for test security (NAN, 2000c) and for copyright protection. It is inappropriate and unethical to make copies of actual tests for patients or other parties as a means of providing feedback on assessment findings (EPPCC; APA, 2002b). Because of the time and expense in properly standardizing psychological and neuropsychological instruments, the clinician is entrusted to safeguard and protect the proprietary aspects of such tests to the fullest degree possible. Test publishers routinely include a section on their recommendations for test security and these should be strictly followed in the best manner possible by each clinician. Unique pressures may arise in certain forensic settings, but again the responsibility of the clinician is to maintain the integrity and security of test materials as far as the law and practice guidelines of psychology apply in the relevant jurisdiction(s) of service or practice. In particular, neuropsychologists are aware of the EPPCC and federal, state, provincial, or local policies that govern the content, security, and release of psychological and neuropsychological reports, test protocols, and raw test data or responses, including mandates from state boards of psychology, the Health Insurance Portability and Accountability Act (HIPAA) and the Centers for Medicare and Medicaid Services (CMS).

D. UNDERSERVED POPULATIONS/CULTURAL ISSUES

The present guidelines augment the "cultural competence" provisions of the EPPCC by defining the issues to be considered and recommending some specific competencies for the neuropsychological evaluation of individuals belonging to minority and underserved populations. Consistent with these provisions, neuropsychologists are aware that cultural, linguistic, disability, and other demographic and socioeconomic factors influence individuals' participation in the process of neuropsychological assessment, and may alter the meaning of the information obtained from testing (see, for example, Artiola i Fortuny et al., 2005; Brauer, 1993; Cohen, Mounty, & Martin, 2005; Manly et al., 1998; Mason, 2005; Ortiz, 2001; Perez-Arce & Puente, 1998; Vernon, 2005; Wong & Fujii, 2004). Neuropsychologists are also aware of the risks inherent in administering and interpreting tests with individuals from groups for whom there are insufficient or limited test adaptations, normative data, or validity studies (see Artiola i Fortuny, Heaton, & Hermosillo, 1998; Manly, 2005). These groups include individuals with unusually low levels of education (in the United States or elsewhere), those whose primary language is other than English and who belong to distinctive cultural or sociodemographic groups, and those with physical or mental disabilities that limit the ability to participate meaningfully in the examination as originally intended.

Neuropsychologists who agree to evaluate members of special populations are specifically educated about issues and have experience in administering and interpreting procedures relevant to the patient in question (Echemendia & Westerveld, 2006; Hauser, Wills, & Isquith, 2006; Ortiz, 2001; Vernon, 2005; Wong & Fujii, 2004). Alternatively, neuropsychologists show (1) that they have sought a local colleague better qualified to accomplish the task, (2) that the potential harm to the patient of deferring or declining the referral has been assessed and is considered to outweigh the potential dangers of proceeding with an evaluation, notwithstanding acknowledged limitations in the neuropsychologist's population-specific competencies, and (3) that they have attempted to ameliorate or compensate for all such limitations by consulting appropriate colleagues and research literature.

Neuropsychologists describe in their report how well they have communicated with the patient, their own level of fluency in the patient's language, and their uncertainty about the fidelity of interpreter-mediated translation and quality of interpersonal communication, including not only literal content, but also culturally mediated meanings, affective tone, and nonverbal "body language." They further note the inevitable effects of using an interpreter on the validity of the test results and interview data (Dean & Pollard, 2005; Glickman & Gulati, 2003; Harvey, Artiola i Fortuny, Vester-Blockland, & De Smedt, 2003; Hindley, Hill, & Bond, 1993; Marcos, 1979). Interpreters are employed in a manner that respects the patient's autonomy and competence (Artiola i Fortuny et al., 2005; Cohen et al., 2005; Dean & Pollard, 2005). Neuropsychologists avoid using family members, friends, or other untrained individuals as interpreters, whenever possible, to preserve patient confidentiality and autonomy as well as to optimize the fidelity of translation.

Neuropsychologists recognize the threats to validity that can occur with the introduction of cultural bias in both translated and adapted instruments. These threats may occur at three levels: item, method, and construct (Van de Vijver & Hambleton, 1996). When working with populations for whom tests have not been standardized and normed, neuropsychologists place particular emphasis on using direct observation and relevant supplementary information about a patient's adaptive functioning within his or her "real-world" community. They may employ assessment strategies that do not require a standardized normative approach, including, but not limited to, direct observation, charting of behavioral changes over time, criterion- referenced testing, direct comparisons with a group of demographically similar peers, or comparison with demographically similar groups in published research studies (Manly, 2005; Simeonsson & Rosenthal, 2001).

6. Methods and Procedures

A. THE DECISION TO EVALUATE

Before initiating neuropsychological testing, the neuropsychologist clarifies the referral source and the referral questions, determines that he or she is competent to evaluate the patient and answer the referral question(s), concludes that it is ethically acceptable to do so, and decides that a neuropsychological evaluation is pertinent to the issues raised. Otherwise, the neuropsychologist contacts the referral source and discusses whether some other type of evaluation may be better to address the referral questions, such as a psychodiagnostic evaluation, functional behavior assessment, clinical interview, psychiatric evaluation or other medical assessment. Alternatively, the neuropsychologist suggests that the evaluation may be more appropriately conducted by a different neuropsychologist owing to conflict of interest or the fit of the patient's needs to the neuropsychologist's clinical competencies or cultural or language expertise.

B. REVIEW OF RECORDS

Having access to information from sources other than the patient and their family members usually allows for a more comprehensive neuropsychological evaluation. Memories may be inaccurate or historical reports distorted, previous information may have been misunderstood or pieced together from the recollections of others, or patients simply may not know important facts. When conducting a comprehensive evaluation, the neuropsychologist attempts to obtain relevant background information from written records whenever possible. By gathering historical information, the neuropsychologist may improve diagnostic predictive accuracy, better describe cognitive and behavioral functioning, and assist treatment planning. In the case of an injury, medical condition, or neurological event, medical records from emergency personnel, hospitals, and outpatient facilities help to establish facts related to the time frame of the presenting problems, presence or absence of critical medical factors, type and degree of injury or impairment, and circumstances under which problems may have become manifest. Historical information is also relevant in assessing patients with histories of psychiatric illness, developmental disabilities, or learning or attentional disorders, and for whom the time sequence of the problems and interventions used to manage these problems may be important in clinical decision making.

In the case of suspected cognitive changes, an attempt to obtain a patient's earlier medical records is advisable in most cases. Although not a common practice in adult neuropsychological assessment, information gathered from available childhood health records helps to determine if pre-existing difficulties may account, in part, for a patient's current level of functioning. In the evaluation of children, adolescents, and young adults, information contained in the school records often enhances understanding of the child's past and current cognitive and behavioral functioning. Records of school or work histories for adults may be similarly useful in providing information on pre-morbid level of functioning, but are often unavailable.

The aims of the evaluation typically determine the extent to which the neuropsychologist gathers information from collateral sources. Extensive review of records may be a worthwhile goal in conducting some assessments, but may not be warranted in all cases and will depend on the nature of the referral questions. In many routine clinical scenarios, such as evaluations undertaken to facilitate ongoing medical care, the patient's best interests may be better served when an interpretive report is provided expeditiously, without the delays that often accompany a request to complete a review of external records. Writing a subsequent addendum summarizing a review of obtained records may be considered as a means to supplement information not available at the time of the original report.

Finally, the nature of the questions asked of a neuropsychologist in a forensic evaluation may require a more extensive review of records than is typically required for a clinical evaluation. In a forensic case, the neuropsychologist reviews as much relevant information about the past and present functioning of the patient as can be made available to him=her. Neuropsychologists do not, when conducting an examination for a forensic purpose, assume primary responsibility for the discovery and production of historical records.

C. Interview of Patient and Significant Others

A neuropsychological evaluation consists of more than a review of records and the administration of psychological and neuropsychological tests. Indeed, some information critical to the evaluation may only be available via a patient interview. Information from the patient may enable the clinician to gain perspective on the patient's experience, including self-perceptions of problems and stresses, and to integrate this information with data from other sources (e.g., test results, record reviews, interviews with significant others). In this way, the clinician may come to a more complete understanding of the patient's history and current situation and be better able to apprehend how the patient or examinee views his=her life circumstances.

Neuropsychologists may employ actuarial (i.e., purely data-driven) approaches to understanding and interpreting brain-behavior relationships, including those that focus solely on lateralization and=or localization of brain dysfunction (Russell, Russell, & Hill, 2005). However, a comprehensive neuropsychological evaluation generally entails identification and description of the cognitive and behavioral correlates of brain disease or neurodevelopmental disorder, opinions regarding prognosis, and formulation of treatment plans. A clinical interview and gathering of historical information, often including neuroimaging or other medical findings, is critical to this process.

When interviewing a patient, the neuropsychologist typically considers the events that led to the referral for an evaluation, the duration of the presenting problems or condition, the primary symptoms and changes in symptom presentation over time, the effect of the presenting symptoms or condition on daily functioning, the results of previously conducted tests and procedures, and the patient's strengths and interests. Relevant historical details may include prenatal history, birth and developmental background, educational history (including any history of learning disabilities or weaknesses), work history, current and past medical and psychiatric history, history of alcohol or substance abuse, current and past medications, legal history, and family medical, psychiatric, and substance abuse history.

Although interviewing a family member or friend of the patient is not always possible, doing so may yield useful information not otherwise available. Because of problems with motivation, memory, language, reduced awareness of their illness, or other neurobehavioral symptoms, patients may not always be reliable informants for past or current events. Information from a person who knows the patient and who can talk about the patient's pre-morbid history, and the effects that the illness=injury has had on the patient and family, can be critical in understanding the functional consequences of the illness=injury. Such individuals may sometimes be the only source of information regarding the onset, clinical course, and magnitude of deficits. However, it is important to communicate to the family or significant other that a doctor-patient relationship does not exist; thus, issues such as confidentiality, release of records, etc., should be discussed in advance. Whether used in evaluating the patient or to obtain information from other informants, a structured interview can help to reduce bias and ensure thoroughness and consistency across examinations. It may also provide a means for standardizing data collection of potential use in clinical research.

D. MEASUREMENT PROCEDURES

Neuropsychological evaluations vary in content depending on their purpose but they typically assess multiple neurocognitive and emotional functions. Primary cognitive domains include: intellectual functions; academic skills (e.g., reading, writing, math); receptive and expressive language skills (e.g., verbal comprehension, fluency, confrontation naming); simple and complex attention; learning and memory (e.g., encoding, recall, recognition); visuospatial abilities; executive functions, problem- solving and reasoning abilities; and sensorimotor skills. Ideally, assessments should also include measures designed to assess personality, social-emotional functioning, and adaptive behavior. In some settings (e.g., testing the acutely medically ill), comprehensive testing may be contra-indicated; in such situations, measurement of selected neurocognitive domains and=or a screening of cognitive skills is preferred. Additional guidelines for test selection can be found in APA's Standards for Educational and Psychological Testing (1999).

Neuropsychological tests and measures used for clinical purposes must meet standards for psychometric adequacy (with exceptions as noted below). These standards include: (1) acceptable levels of reliability, (2) demonstrated validity in relation to other tests and=or to brain status, including evidence that the test or measure assesses the process, ability, or trait it purports to assess, and (3) normative standards that allow the clinician to evaluate the patient's scores in relation to relevant patient characteristics, such as age, gender, and sociodemographic or cultural=linguistic background. In general, tests published with large, stratified normative samples—"Heaton norms" (Heaton, Avitabile, Grant, & Matthews, 1999); Mayo's Older Americans Normative Studies (MOANS; Ivnik et al., 1992, 1996), and Mayo's Older African Americans Normative Studies (MOAANS; Lucas et al., 2005)—provide a sound foundation for accurate interpretation. Comparisons of results from tests that are co-normed are advantageous in examining differences between two or more cognitive domains. The neuropsychologist is aware of the source of normative data and is cautious about using tests for which sample sizes are small or restricted (e.g., by geographic region or sociodemographic characteristics). Sample size considerations are particularly important in child assessments, where developmental changes in skills demand adequate sampling across a variety of ages.

Measures that show promise, but have not met the most rigorous standards, may be considered to assess skills, behaviors, or influences that are deemed important to elucidate patients' or others' concerns. However, these more "provisional" tests and measures are selected to complement rather than replace those with better-established properties. Preliminary evidence for psychometric adequacy is needed even for measures considered provisional in nature; and the neuropsychologist is aware of the level of support for their use in interpreting the findings.

Some common conditions that justify exceptions to the general principles elucidated above include: the need to evaluate an individual whose neuropsychological functioning falls at the extremes of the normal distribution (e.g., those with mental retardation or the exceptionally gifted), individuals with sensory or motor disabilities that require modifications to standardized test administration (e.g., creating a bedside assessment for a patient with neglect following a right hemisphere stroke), and individuals from linguistic or cultural groups for whom no normed test exists. In such cases, the neuropsychologist recognizes the importance of ecologic validity or external "real-world" validation of the test findings and for determining the reliability of the findings across multiple tests. The neuropsychologist also explicitly acknowledges in the report the modifications of test administration and scoring and their potential effect on the validity of the assessment results.

A comprehensive neuropsychological evaluation should be thorough but also efficient and respectful of a patient's time and resources. Some patients, such as those who fatigue easily, may require more than one session. Furthermore, in clinical practice, clinical neuropsychologists often find it necessary and advisable to administer a selected set of subtests instead of the complete test battery or test. An advantage of using multiple tests from single or co-normed test batteries is that patient strengths and weaknesses, including levels or laterality of performance, can be assessed relative to the same normative sample. A further advantage is that administration of test batteries can provide for the assessment of a broad range of functions. Disadvantages include a predetermined number and restricted selection of subtests in the existing test batteries, and associated time constraints, which may preclude administration of complete batteries when given in combination with other measures of interest. Breadth of assessment can be provided by administering multiple individual tests and=or combinations of subtests from different test batteries, depending on the goals of the evaluation. The practice of using selected subtests or individually developed tests can be justified by reference to research literature employing these measures and the availability of appropriate normative standards (e.g., Baron, 2004; Heaton et al., 1999; Lucas et al., 2005; Steinberg & Bieliauskas, 2005).

E. ASSESSMENT OF MOTIVATION AND EFFORT

A growing literature suggests that the assessment of motivation and effort is critical when conducting a neuropsychological evaluation (Bush & NAN Policy & Planning Committee, 2005b). This area has received the greatest emphasis in forensic assessment, in which symptom magnification, impression management, or even feigning of impairment can occur (Mittenberg, Patton, Canyock, & Condit, 2002). However, the assessment of effort and motivation is important in any clinical setting, as a patient's effort may be compromised even in the absence of any potential or active litigation, compensation, or financial incentives. Approaches for assessing motivation and effort include: behavioral observations from interview or testing of behaviors such as avoidance, resistance, hostility, and lack of cooperation; examination of the pattern of performance among traditional neuropsychological measures; identification of unexpected or unusually slow and=or impaired levels of performance; identification of cognitive profiles that do not fit with known patterns typical of brain disorders; and consideration of suspect performance on objective measures of effort. Clinicians utilize multiple indicators of effort, including tasks and paradigms validated for this purpose, to ensure that decisions regarding adequacy of effort are based on converging evidence from several sources, rather than depending on a single measure or method.

Neuropsychologists utilize commonsense methods to optimize patient performance, such as attending to the lighting, seating, and other aspects of physical comfort during testing; treating patients respectfully; establishing rapport; asking the patient about his=her understanding and acceptance of the evaluation process; and encouraging and reinforcing effort. The purpose of these methods is to establish a physically and interpersonally comfortable testing environment, with the goal of minimizing anxiety, resistance, physical discomfort, or other factors that may interfere with optimal motivation and effort.

F. ASSESSMENT OF CONCURRENT VALIDITY

The neuropsychologist typically draws inferences about a given skill or ability from more than one test or test score, and considers the influences of the patient's state of engagement, arousal, or fatigue on test performance. To illustrate, issues of test validity may be raised when performance on an attention measure early in a test battery is better than performance on another attention task toward the end of the battery. Cultural and language-mediated effects on test performance are also considered, and caution is exercised in administering and interpreting tests to individuals from a demographic, linguistic, or cultural group for which the tests have not been appropriately normed, validated, and translated (see section 5C). The neuropsychologist should be aware of limitations of making comparisons among standard scores arising from different normative samples and should make efforts to include norms that are most similar to the demographics of the patient being examined.

G. TEST ADMINISTRATION AND SCORING

Standard procedures are followed in test administration and scoring (see Standards for Educational and Psychological Testing, APA, 1999). Tests are administered, scored, and interpreted in ways that are consistent with evidence regarding the utility and appropriate application of these methods. The clinician attempts to prevent misuse of the test materials, and to determine and report circumstances in which norms may have limited applicability or test procedures may be inapplicable or require modification (EPPCC). Neuropsychologists may "test limits" (e.g., by changing test demands or providing extra time) to investigate the effects of accommodations on test performance, but findings from such procedures are clearly labeled as such and norms that apply to standard administrations are not used to describe the results. The presence of third-party observers during test administration is also strongly discouraged (AACN, 2001; NAN, 2000a). If a third party or monitoring device is present, the neuropsychologist states how and to what extent this circumstance may have affected the test results.

Accuracy of scoring is essential for appropriate interpretation of test results. The neuropsychologist is familiar with scoring methods and criteria for specific items, procedures for aggregating scores, and the meaning of the scores (i.e., the normative base used for converting raw to standard, or derived scores). Scoring is performed with care, with double-checking of scores, sums, and conversion tables to ensure accuracy. If novel scoring procedures are used, they should be justified by previous research. Computer scoring programs, because of the "hidden" nature of their operations, are used only if validated against other reliable and previously validated procedures. Neuropsychologists are responsible for the accuracy of scores when a psychometrist or computerized scoring program are utilized (APA, 1992; NAN, 2000b).

H. INTERPRETATION

Accurate interpretation of neuropsychological test data requires extensive relevant training and experience, and knowledge of current empirically based professional opinions gathered from continuing education and the published literature. A neuropsychologist's clinical interpretation of the evaluation findings is based on information regarding the patient's history and problems, direct observation of the patient, levels or patterns of test performance associated with specific clinical presentations, and the current theory and knowledge regarding the neurological and psychosocial=cultural influences on test performance and daily functioning. This interpretation is highly individualized and does not follow a "cookbook" approach. Results from computer scoring and interpretation programs are also considered within the context of the individual patient; the neuropsychologist does not exclusively use automated computer printout interpretation as a substitute for a carefully considered and individually tailored clinical interpretation.

Information about the patient's sociodemographic status, cultural and linguistic background, and work, school, and family characteristics can be obtained through interview or formal measures. These factors are taken into consideration in making judgments as to the extent to which the test performance deviates from expected levels (see section 5C). This information is also useful in determining if environmental or motivational factors are contributing to or exacerbating the patient's problems.

The inferences made by neuropsychologists in interpreting the evaluation findings include judgments regarding: (1) the nature of the cognitive deficits or patterns of strengths and weaknesses, (2) the likely sources of, or contributors to, these deficits or patterns, and (3) their relation to the patient's presenting problems and implications for treatment and prognosis. The first type of inference is based on knowledge of the cognitive constructs measured by neuropsychological tests. Judgments regarding relative strengths and weaknesses also rely on knowledge of expected levels of test performance relative to background patient characteristics or to the patient's performance on other tests (as in making judgments regarding inter-test score discrepancies). In rendering conclusions regarding a patient's strengths and weaknesses, the clinician considers the consistency of findings across multiple tests and alternative explanations for high or low test scores (e.g., development of compensatory test-taking strategies, poor effort) or the overall pattern and profile of neuropsychological test scores.

The second type of inference, regarding causal or contributing factors, relies on knowledge of the cognitive, behavioral, and emotional consequences of brain insults or constitutional-genetic anomalies. If a brain insult or neurodevelopmental anomaly is known, a judgment is made as to whether the insult or anomaly has contributed in some way to the patient's problems. The insult or anomaly may be a primary cause of the problems. In circumstances in which several causal factors are potentially contributory, it may be difficult to conclude with reasonable certainty that a particular event or disease is the primary cause, or to isolate the specific influence of a particular condition on a behavior or learning problem. Inferences regarding causation take into account not only the pattern of the test results, but also the history of the patient's problems, the nature of the potential causal event and its relation to symptom presentation, the strength of research supporting a relation between the type of brain insult or anomaly of the patient and the test findings, the base rate of the problem in the general population, and alternative explanations for the patient's test findings. These same considerations apply if the brain insult or anomaly is unknown. In this latter instance, the judgment to be made involves the extent to which the problems are consistent with or suggest the presence, nature, or localization of a neurological abnormality. Inferences in this regard are again based on the degree of consistency of the patient's test results to those of other patients with similar insults or anomalies, the likelihood of a neurological insult or anomaly as having occurred, the patient's history and timing of symptoms in relation to a potential insult or anomaly, and consideration of other possible causes for the patient's problems.

In making judgments regarding brain insult or anomaly as a cause for the patient's presenting problems, co-morbidities, or ability deficits, the neuropsychologist considers factors that may ameliorate or exacerbate these effects. Such moderating variables may include patient behavior and background characteristics, environmental supports or stressors, the effects of various medications, and the patient's current level of cognitive functioning.

Environmental and maturational influences on outcomes of brain insult or anomaly are also considered in making judgments regarding causation.

The third type of inference pertains to the validity of neuropsychological test results in identifying and forecasting social-behavioral or learning problems and in predicting responsiveness to different interventions. Test validity in this sense is supported to the extent that the patient's identified deficits, or patterns of strengths and weaknesses, have been related in past research to problems similar to the patient's. Further support for validity comes from studies indicating that specific deficits or patterns of strengths and weaknesses predict other difficulties or future outcomes, or inform treatment for the patient's problems. In drawing conclusions about the relevance of cognitive skills to identification and management of a patient's problems, the neuropsychologist considers the possible contributions of non-cognitive factors (e.g., the effects of pain, sleep disruption, medication effects, psychological distress or history of maladaptive behavior unrelated to the patient's cognitive deficits, social or educational supports).

New technologies for evaluating brain–behavior relationships are emerging, including advances in neuroimaging, genetic analyses, metabolic tests, and other measures that reflect physiological and psychological functions. All of the major areas of clinical psychometric assessment, as defined earlier in these guidelines, are being standardized for research and clinical purposes using an array of neuroimaging methods, such as functional magnetic resonance imaging (fMRI). To illustrate, APA Division 40 has endorsed the role of neuropsychologists in clinical use of fMRI (APA, 2004). In the coming years, standardized assessment protocols for assessing a broad spectrum of neuropsychiatric and cognitive disorders are likely to be developed wherein clinical neuropsychologists will use neuroimaging as part of their neuropsychological evaluation and assessment.

I. THE EVALUATION REPORT

Neuropsychological findings generally are summarized in a written report to be provided to the referral source or responsible party (Axelrod, 1999), except in special circumstances (e.g., certain forensic or research contexts). The EPPCC (APA, 2002b, 6.01: Documentation of Professional and Scientific Work) notes that the written report serves "... to facilitate provision of services later; to ensure accountability; and to meet other requirements of institutions or the law."

Report writing styles vary with the purpose of the report, background and training of the neuropsychologist, requirements of the work setting, and even, on occasion, the specific guidelines established by the referring party. Neuropsychological evaluations are typically requested for a specific purpose or to answer specific referral questions. The purposes of the assessment may include provision of differential diagnoses, documentation of cognitive strengths and weaknesses, delineation of functional implications of the identified deficits, and recommendations regarding interventions. Generally speaking, the aims of the report are (1) to describe the patient and record the findings, (2) to interpret the patient's performance on tests in light of other assessment information, (3) to answer questions and make judgments regarding the nature and sources of the presenting complaints=concerns, (4) to assess prognosis and make recommendations for future care, and (5) to communicate the results to the patient or significant others with permission, to the referral source, and other service providers such as teachers and therapists (Axelrod, 1999).

Despite the absence of a universally accepted outline or format, the report usually is organized to assist the reader in identifying the patient and learning of the reason for referral and presenting problems, the patient's history and level of functioning, the patient's behavior during the evaluation, the test results, and the clinician's impressions, interpretations, and recommendations. Some of the most commonly used report sections include: Identifying Information and Reason for Referral; Background Information=History; Tests Administered; Behavioral Observations; Test Results=Interpretations; Summary & Conclusions; Diagnostic Impressions; and Recommendations. Consultations or short reports are more annotated versions of the above format, typically consisting of a few paragraphs describing the test results and recommendations. Abbreviated reports are more common when evaluating patients whose background is already known to the referral source (e.g., primary physician) or when the assessment is being conducted for more circumscribed reasons (e.g., to assess cognitive function as part of a multidisciplinary inpatient assessment). Test reports contain information regarding the patient's age, gender, educational level, occupational background, need for special services or accommodations in conducting the assessment, racial identity=ethnicity, the persons who conducted the assessment (neuropsychologist, psychometrist) and others present during testing (e.g., translator, student trainee), and (as appropriate) the language(s) in which testing was conducted and the examiner's and patient's fluency in the language(s).

One recommended practice in clinical neuropsychology is to include numerical data (including scaled scores or percentile ranks) in reports (Donders, 2001; Friedes, 1993). Neuropsychologists may choose to append test scores in a summary sheet, or insert scores in the report text. Including test scores allows for the comparison of a patient's performance over repeated evaluations, minimizes the need for obtaining multiple releases of information, and increases the efficiency with which raw data can be shared with other professionals for the purpose of further assessment or management of the patient. Inclusion of scores also increases accountability and may even minimize and clarify any interpretation biases or idiosyncrasies on the part of the writer (Matarazzo, 1995). Finally, in certain situations, such as documenting a learning disability or ADHD for higher education, the guidelines issued by testing organizations and used by academic institutions universally require the reporting of test scores (Educational Testing Service (1998a, 1998b). When used in conjunction with scores, use of words describing test scores (e.g., "below average," "impaired") may facilitate understanding of test data.

Multiple normative data sets are available for many neuropsychological instruments, and test score percentiles or standard scores may differ depending on which norms are employed. As appropriate, citations may be provided for the normative sets, which can assist the reader in understanding how specific standard scores were derived. Further, because some test norms allow adjustment for age, while others also correct for additional factors, such as education, gender, and=or ethnicity, some practitioners may choose to specify the demographic characteristics that were considered in deriving norm-based scores (e.g., 10th percentile for age and education; Selnes et al., 1991).

J. PROVIDING FEEDBACK

Although documentation of the results from a neuropsychological evaluation usually takes the form of a written summary or report, feedback is often provided directly (i.e., in a face-to-face meeting or phone call) to referral sources, patients, families, third-party payers, and the legal system. Feedback to clinical referral sources is provided in a timely manner and addresses the relevant referral questions and concerns. The neuropsychologist also makes additional inferences and recommendations as appropriate for the benefit of the patient or referral source. For example, the need for patient counseling or special school placements may be advised, even if questions regarding these matters were not raised by the referral source.

Feedback regarding the evaluation findings and recommendations are provided in a manner that is comprehensible to intended recipients and which respects the well-being, dignity, and rights of the individual examinee. Ethical and legal guidelines pertaining to the provision of feedback should be identified and followed. As noted earlier (section 5B), feedback typically is not given in forensic evaluations, but it is part of most clinical evaluations. The neuropsychologist adheres to professional ethics (EPPCC) and federal, state, and local laws related to the autonomy and decision-making capacities of patients who are legally competent. When cognitive impairments interfere with the patient's ability to understand the implications of the test results, or in the case of a child examinee, feedback may be provided to a responsible party (legal guardian or parent), with or without the patient present. The neuropsychologist consults with the responsible party to decide whether or not to provide direct feedback to a minor child or vulnerable adult. In some such cases, sensitive and developmentally appropriate discussion of results and recommendations may enhance the person's well-being; in other cases, direct feedback about test findings could be detrimental, particularly if the child or vulnerable adult misconstrues what is said.

References

American Academy of Clinical Neuropsychology. (2001). Policy statement on the presence of third party observers in neuropsychological assessments. *The Clinical Neuropsychologist*, 15, 433–439.

American Psychological Association. (1992). Official position of the division of clinical neuropsychology (APA division 40) regarding the use of nondoctoral personnel for neuropsychological assessment. *The Clinical Neuropsychologist*, 6, 256.

American Psychological Association. (1999). *Standards for educational and psychological testing*. Washington, DC: APA.

American Psychological Association. (2002a). Criteria for practice guideline development and evaluation. *American Psychologist*, 57, 1048–1051.

American Psychological Association. (2002b). Ethical principles of psychologists and code of conduct. *American Psychologist*, 57, 1060–1073.

American Psychological Association. (2004). Official position of the division of clinical neuropsychology (APA division 40) on the role of neuropsychologists in clinical use of fMRI. *The Clinical Neuropsychologist*, 18, 349–351.

American Psychological Association. (2005). Determination and documentation of the need for practice guidelines. *American Psychologist*, 60, 976–978.

American Psychological Association. (2006). Evidence-based practice in psychology. *American Psychologist*, 61, 271–283.

Artiola i Fortuny, L., Garolera, M., Hermosillo Romo, D., Feldman, E., Fernandez Barillas, H., Keefe, R. et al. (2005). Research with Spanish-speaking populations in the United

States: Lost in the translation. A commentary and a plea. *Journal of the International Neuropsychological Society, 27,* 555–564.

Artiola i Fortuny, L., Heaton, R. K., & Hermosillo, D. (1998). Neuropsychological comparisons of Spanish-speaking participants from the U.S.–Mexico border region versus Spain. *Journal of the International Neuropsychological Society, 4,* 363–379.

Axelrod, B. N. (1999). Neuropsychological report writing. In R. D. Vanderploeg (Ed.), *Clinician's guide to neuropsychological assessment.* Hillsdale, NJ: Lawrence Erlbaum.

Baron, I. S. (2004). *Neuropsychological evaluation of the child.* New York: Oxford University Press.

Barth, J. T., Pliskin, N., Axelrod, B., Faust, D., Fisher, J., Harley, J. P. et al. (2003). Introduction to the NAN 2001 definition of a clinical neuropsychologist. NAN policy and planning committee. *Archives of Clinical Neuropsychology, 18,* 551–555.

Bieliauskas, L. A. (1999). Mediocrity is no standard: Searching for self-respect in clinical neuropsychology. *The Clinical Neuropsychologist, 13,* 1–11.

Bornstein, R. A. (1988a). Entry into clinical neuropsychology: Graduate, undergraduate and beyond. *The Clinical Neuropsychologist, 2,* 213–220.

Bornstein, R. A. (1988b). Reports of the division 40 task force on education, accreditation and credentialing. *The Clinical Neuropsychologist, 2,* 25–29.

Brauer, B. A. (1993). Adequacy of a translation of the MMPI into American sign language for use with deaf individuals: Linguistic equivalency issues. *Rehabilitation Psychology, 38,* 247–260.

Bush, S. S. & the NAN Policy & Planning Committee. (2005a). Independent and court ordered forensic neuropsychological examinations: Official statement of the national academy of neuropsychology. *Archives of Clinical Neuropsychology, 20,* 997–1007.

Bush, S. S. & the NAN Policy & Planning Committee. (2005b). Symptom validity assessment: Practice issues and medical necessity: Official statement of the national academy of neuropsychology. *Archives of Clinical Neuropsychology, 20,* 419–426.

Cohen, O., Mounty, J., & Martin, D. (2005). *Assessing Deaf adults: Critical issues in testing and evaluation.* Washington, DC: Gallaudet University Press.

Cripe, L. (2000). Division 40 special presentation: Listing of training programs in clinical neuropsychology–2000. *The Clinical Neuropsychologist, 14,* 357–448.

Dean, R. & Pollard, R. (2005). Consumers and service effectiveness in interpreting work: A practice profession perspective. In M. Marschark, R. Peterson, & W. Winston (Eds.), *Interpreting and interpreter education: Directions for research and practice* (pp. 259–282). New York: Oxford University Press.

Donders, J. (2001). A survey of report writing by neuropsychologists, II: Test data, report format, and document length. *The Clinical Neuropsychologist, 15,* 150–161.

Donders, J. (2002). Survey of graduates of programs affiliated with the association of postdoctoral programs in clinical neuropsychology (APPCN). *The Clinical Neuropsychologist, 16,* 413–425.

Echemendia, R. & Westerveld, M. (2006). Cultural considerations in pediatric rehabilitation. In J. Farmer, J. Donders, & S. Warschausky (Eds.), *Treating neurodevelopmental disorders.* New York: Guilford Press.

Educational Testing Service. (1998a). *Policy statement for documentation of a learning disability in adolescents and adults.* Princeton, NJ: ETS.

Educational Testing Service. (1998b). *Policy statement for documentation of attention-deficit hyperactivity disorder (ADHD) in adolescents and adults.* Princeton, NJ: ETS.

Freides, D. (1993). Proposed standard of professional practice: Neuropsychological reports display all quantitative data. *The Clinical Neuropsychologist, 7*, 234–235.

Glickman, N. & Gulati, S. (2003). *Mental health care of deaf people: A culturally affirmative approach.* Mahwah, NJ: Lawrence Erlbaum Associates Inc.

Hannay, H. J., Bieliauskas, L. A., Crosson, B. A., Hammeke, T. A., Hamsher, K.deS., & Koffler, S. P. (1998). Proceedings of the Houston Conference on specialty education and training in clinical neuropsychology. *Archives of Clinical Neuropsychology, 13*, 157–158.

Harvey, P. D., Artiola i Fortuny, L., Vester-Blockland, E., & De Smedt, G. (2003). Crossnational cognitive assessment in schizophrenia clinical trials: A feasibility study. *Schizophrenia Research, 59*, 243–251.

Hauser, P., Wills, K. E., & Isquith, P. (2006). Hard of hearing, deafness, and being deaf. In J. Farmer, J. Donders, & S. Warschausky (Eds.), *Treating neurodevelopmental disorders.* New York: Guilford Press.

Heaton, R. K., Avitable, N., Grant, I., & Matthews, C. G. (1999). Further cross validation of regression-based neuropsychological norms with an update for the boston naming test. *Journal of Clinical and Experimental Neuropsychology, 21*, 572–582.

Hindley, P., Hill, P., & Bond, D. (1993). Interviewing deaf children, the interviewer effect: A research note. *Journal of Child Psychology and Psychiatry, 34*, 1461–1467.

Ivnik, R. J., Malec, J. F., Smith, G. E., Tangalos, E. G., Peterson, R. C., Kokmen, E., et al. (1992). Mayo's older American normative studies: WAIS-R, WMS-R and AVLT norms for ages 56 through 97. *The Clinical Neuropsychologist, 6*(Suppl.), 1–104.

Ivnik, R. J., Malec, J. F., Smith, G. E., Tangalos, E. G., & Peterson, R. C. (1996). Neuropsychological tests' norms above age 55: COWAT, BNT < MAE, Token, WRAT-R Reading, AMNART, STROOP, TMT and JLO. *The Clinical Neuropsychologist, 10*, 262–278.

Johnson-Green, D. & the NAN Policy & Planning Committee. (2005). Informed consent in clinical neuropsychology practice: Official statement of the national academy of neuropsychology. *Archives of Clinical Neuropsychology, 20*, 335–340.

Kane, R. L., Goldstein, G., & Parsons, O. A. (1989). A response to Mapou. *Journal of Clinical and Experimental Neuropsychology, 11*, 589–595.

Lamberty, G. J., Courtney, J., & Heilbronner, R. L. (Eds.). (2003), *The practice of clinical neuropsychology.* Lisse: Swets & Zeitlinger.

Lezak, M. D., Howieson, D., & Loring, D. (2004). *Neuropsychological assessment (4th ed.).* New York: Oxford University Press.

Lucas, J. A., Ivnik, R. J., Willis, F. B., Ferman, T. J., Smith, G. E., Parfitt, F. C. et al. (2005). Mayo's older African Americans normative studies: Normative data for commonly used clinical neuropsychological measures. *The Clinical Neuropsychologist, 19*, 162–183.

Manly, J. J. (2005). Advantages and disadvantages of separate norms for African Americans. *The Clinical Neuropsychologist, 19*, 270–275.

Manly, J. J., Miller, S. W., Heaton, R. K., Byrd, D., Reilly, J., Velasquez, R. J. et al. (1998). The effect of African-American acculturation on neuropsychological test performance in normal and HIV-positive individuals. The HIV neurobehavioral research center (HNRC) group. *Journal of the International Neuropsychological Society, 4*, 291–302.

Marcos, L. R. (1979). Effects of interpreters on the evaluation of psychopathology in non-English speaking patients. *American Journal of Psychiatry, 136*, 171–174.

Mason, T. (2005). Cross cultural instrument translation: Assessment, translation, and statistical applications. *American Annals of the Deaf, 150*, 67–72.

Matarazzo, J. D. (1990). Psychological assessment versus psychological testing: Validation from binet to the school, clinic, and courtroom. *American Psychologist, 45,* 999–1017.

Matarazzo, R. G. (1995). Psychological report standards in neuropsychology. *The Clinical Neuropsychologist, 9,* 249–250.

Meyer, G. J., Finn, S. E., Eyde, L. D., Moreland, K. L., Dies, R. R., Eisman, E. J. et al. (2001). Psychological testing and psychological assessment: A review of evidence and issues. *American Psychologist, 56,* 128–165.

Mittenberg, W., Patton, C., Canyock, E. M., & Condit, D. C. (2002). Baserates of malingering and symptom exaggeration. *Journal of Clinical and Experimental Neuropsychology, 24,* 1094–1102.

National Academy of Neuropsychology. (2000a). Presence of third party observers during neuropsychological testing: Official statement of the National Academy of Neuropsychology. *Archives of Clinical Neuropsychology, 15,* 379–380.

National Academy of Neuropsychology. (2000b). The use of neuropsychology test technicians in clinical practice. Official statement of the National Academy of Neuropsychology. *Archives of Clinical Neuropsychology, 15,* 381–382.

National Academy of Neuropsychology. (2000c). Test security: Official statement of the National Academy of Neuropsychology. *Archives of Clinical Neuropsychology, 15,* 383–386.

National Academy of Neuropsychology. (2001). Definition of a clinical neuropsychologist. *Archives of Clinical Neuropsychology, 18,* 551–555.

Ortiz, S. O. (2001). Assessment of cognitive abilities in Hispanic children. *Seminars in Speech and Language, 22,* 17–36.

Perez-Arce, P. & Puente, A. (1998). Neuropsychological assessment of ethnic minorities: The case of assessing hispanics living in North America. In R. J. Sbordone & C. J. Long (Eds.), *Ecological validity of neuropsychological testing* (pp. 283–300). Delray Beach, FL: St. Lucie Press.

Prigatano, G. P. (2002). Neuropsychology, the patient's experience, and the political forces within our field–The problem of lost normality after brain injury. *Archives of Clinical Neuropsychology, 15,* 71–82.

Prigatano, G. P. & Pliskin, N. H. (2003). *Clinical neuropsychology and cost outcome research.* New York: Psychology Press.

Rourke, B. P. & Murji, S. (2000). A history of the international neuropsychological society: The early years (1965–1985). *Journal of the International Neuropsychological Society, 6,* 491–509.

Russell, E. W., Russell, S. L. K., & Hill, B. D. (2005). The fundamental psychometric status of neuropsychological batteries. *Archives of Clinical Neuropsychology, 20,* 785–794.

Selnes, O. A., Jacobson, L., Machado, A. M., Becker, J. T., Wesch, J., Miller, E. N. et al. (1991). Normative data for a brief neuropsychological screening battery. Multicenter AIDS cohort study. *Perceptual and Motor Skills, 73,* 539–550.

Simeonsson, R. & Rosenthal, S. (Eds.). (2001). *Psychological and developmental assessment: Children with disabilities and chronic conditions.* New York: Guilford Press.

Sweet, J. J., Peck, E., Abramowitz, C., & Etzweiler, S. (2000). National academy of neuropsychology/division 40 of the American psychological association practice survey of clinical neuropsychology in the United States, Part I: Practitioner and practice characteristics, professional activities, and time requirements. *The Clinical Neuropsychologist, 16,* 109–127.

Van de Vijver, F. & Hambleton, R. K. (1996). Translating tests: Some practical guidelines. *European Psychologist, 1*, 89–99.

Vanderploeg, R. D. (Ed.). (2000). *Clinician's guide to neuropsychological assessment.* Mahwah, NJ: Lawrence Erlbaum Associates Inc.

Vernon, M. (2005). Fifty years of research on the intelligence of deaf and hard-of-hearing children: A review of literature and discussion of implications. *Journal of Deaf Studies and Deaf Education, 10*, 225–231.

Wong, T. M. & Fujii, D. E. (2004). Neuropsychological assessment of Asian Americans: Demographic factors, cultural diversity, and practical guidelines. *Applied Neuropsychology, 11*, 23–36.

Background of the Guideline Development Process

At its June 2003 annual meeting in Minneapolis, AACN sponsored a forum chaired by Robert Heilbronner to discuss the need for and feasibility of developing practice guidelines for neuropsychology. There was general support for considering this project, with due circumspection, and there were no dissenting opinions. Subsequently, noting that such a project was consistent with its mission and bylaws, the AACN Board of Directors approved the formation of a Practice Guidelines Working Group under the auspices of its Practice Committee, initially co-chaired by Robert Heilbronner and Michael Schmidt. Beginning in 2004, following Dr. Schmidt's resignation, the group was chaired by Dr. Heilbronner.

The working group was assembled from AACN members by invitation of the co-chairs, to include individuals who would provide broad representation in the field of neuropsychology. The group included neuropsychologists who work in a variety of settings, including independent practice, clinics, hospitals, and universities (see list of practice guidelines subcommittee members, below). Professional emphases encompassed the adult, child, forensic, and research arenas. The group included individuals who had held elected offices in various neuropsychological organizations and who had served on the editorial boards of a number of professional journals. The co-chairs assembled a packet of core references, including a number of published position papers relevant to the practice of clinical neuropsychology, as well as policy statements and ethical guidelines of APA and other scientific and professional organizations. The references were provided to each working group member. In addition, individual working group members used their professional judgment and discretion in considering the professional literature within their areas of expertise.

An initial working group meeting was held during the 2004 INS meeting in Baltimore. A general outline of the guidelines was approved, and group members volunteered to take primary responsibility for portions of this outline based on their specific areas of interest and expertise. To ensure a broader perspective, at least two individuals were assigned to each area. Initial drafts were compiled, and revisions were made based on input from all working group members.

The committee met again in St. Louis at the 2005 INS Meeting and further revisions were made. After that meeting, the draft document, including literature citations, was approved by a general consensus from working group members. The document was then submitted to an independent peer-review panel of senior neuropsychologists for comments (see senior level peer-reviewers, below). Following further revisions based on this review, a revised document was submitted to the AACN board and reviewed first by the President (R. Mapou) and Vice-President (J. Sweet). Revisions were recommended and made by Dr. Heilbronner and selected group members. The document was submitted to the board on November 15, 2005, where it was reviewed by all members of the board of directors.

Consolidated comments were provided from the board to the Practice Guidelines Committee on January 7, 2006. A number of revisions and changes were recommended. These were made and a final document was submitted to the board on May 1, 2006. It was reviewed by all members of the board and accepted in its current form on June 16, 2006.

Practice Guidelines Subcommittee

Robert L. Heilbronner (chair), H. Gerry Taylor, Karen Wills, Kyle Boone, Erin Bigler, Lidia Artiola i Fortuny, Neil H. Pliskin, Richard F. Kaplan, Greg Lamberty, and Michael Schmidt.

Senior Level Peer-Reviewers

Ken Adams (chair), Carl Dodrill, Wilfred van Gorp, and Ida Sue Baron.

Allott, K. & Lloyd, S. (2009). The provision of neuropsychological services in rural/regional settings: Professional and ethical issues. *Applied Neuropsychology, 16*(3), 193–206.

Allport, G. W. (1961). *Pattern and growth in personality.* New York: Holt, Rinehart, & Winston.

American Academy of Clinical Neuropsychology (AACN, 1999). AACN policy on the use of non-doctoral-level personnel in conducting clinical neuropsychological evaluations. *The Clinical Neuropsychologist, 13*(4), 385.

American Academy of Clinical Neuropsychology (2001). Policy statement on the presence of third party observers in neuropsychological assessments. *The Clinical Neuropsychologist, 15*(4), 433–439.

American Psychological Association (2002). Ethical principles of psychologists and code of conduct. *American Psychologist, 57* (12), 1060–1073.

American Psychological Association (APA, 2004). Official position of the division of clinical neuropsychology (APA Division 40) on the role of neuropsychologists in clinical use of fMRI: Approved by the Division 40 executive committee July 28, 2004. *The Clinical Neuropsychologist, 18*(3), 349–351.

American Psychological Association Commission for the Recognition of Specialties and Proficiencies in Professional Psychology. (2010). *Public description of clinical neuropsychology.* Downloaded November 21, 2010, from http://www.apa.org/ed/graduate/specialize/neuro.aspx.

American Psychological Association. (2006). Evidence-based practice in psychology. *American Psychologist, 61*(4), 271–283.

Anson, K., & Ponsford, J. (2006). Evaluation of a coping skills group following traumatic brain injury. *Brain Injury, 20*(2), 167–178.

Ardila, A. (2002). Houston conference: Need for more fundamental knowledge in neuropsychology. *Neuropsychology Review, 12*(3), 127–130.

Armstrong, K., Beebe, D. W., Hilsabeck, R. C., & Kirkwood, M. W. (2008). *Board certification in clinical neuropsychology: A guide to becoming ABPP/ABCN certified without sacrificing your sanity.* New York: Oxford University Press.

Arnold, G., Boone, K. B., Lu, P., Dean, A., Wen, J., Nitch, S. & McPherson, S. (2005). Sensitivity and specificity of finger tapping test scores for the detection of suspect effort. *The Clinical Neuropsychologist, 19*(1), 105–120.

Artiola i Fortuny, L. (2008). Research and practice: Ethical issues with immigrant adults and children. In J. E. Morgan & J. H. Ricker (Eds.), *Textbook of Clinical Neuropsychology* (pp. 960–981). New York: Taylor & Francis.

Attix, D. K., Donders, J., Johnson-Greene, D., Grote, C. L., Harris, J. G., & Bauer, R. M. (2007). Disclosure of neuropsychological test data: Official position of division 40 (clinical neuropsychology) of the American Psychological Association, Association of Postdoctoral Programs in Clinical Neuropsychology, and American Academy of Clinical Neuropsychology. *The Clinical Neuropsychologist, 21*(2), 232–238.

Attix, D. K. & Potter, G. G. (2010). Increasing awareness of clinical neuropsychology in the general public. *The Clinical Neuropsychologist, 24*(3), 391–400.

Axelrod, B. N. (2000). Neuropsychological report writing. In R. D. Vanderploeg (Ed.), *Clinician's guide to neuropsychological assessment*, 2nd ed. (pp. 245–273). Mahwah, NJ: Erlbaum.

Axelrod, B., Heilbronner, R., Barth, J., Larrabee, G., Faust, D., Pliskin, N., et al. (2000). Test security: Official position statement of the National Academy of Neuropsychology. *Archives of Clinical Neuropsychology, 15*(5), 383–386.

Bailey, K. M., Carleton, R. N., Vlaeyen, J. W. S., & Asmundson, G. J. G. (2010). Treatments addressing pain-related fear and anxiety in patients with chronic musculoskeletal pain: A preliminary review. *Cognitive Behaviour Therapy, 39*(1), 46–63.

Barona, A., Reynolds, C. R., & Chastain, R. (1984). A demographically based index of pre-morbid intelligence for the WAIS-R. *Journal of Consulting and Clinical Psychology, 52*(5), 885–887.

Barr, W. B. (2008). Historical development of the neuropsychological test battery. in J. E. Morgan & J. H. Ricker (Eds.), *Textbook of clinical neuropsychology. Studies on neuropsychology, neurology and cognition.* New York: Psychology Press.

Beck, A. T., Steer, R. A., & Brown, G. K. (1996). *Beck Depression Inventory (2nd ed.).* San Antonio, TX: The Psychological Corporation.

Benedict, R. H. B. (1997). *Brief Visuospatial Memory Test–Revised.* Odessa, FL: Psychological Assessment Resources.

Benton, A. L. (2000). *Exploring the history of neuropsychology: selected papers.* New York: Oxford University Press.

Benton, A. L., Hamsher, K. de S., Rey, G. J., & Sivan, A. B. (1994). *Multilingual Aphasia Examination (3rd ed.).* Iowa City, IA: AJA Associates.

Benton, A. L., Sivan, a. B., Hamsher, K. deS., Varney, N. R., & Spreen, O. (1994). *Contributions to neuropsychological assessment (2nd ed.).* Orlando, FL: Psychological Assessment Resources.

Berry, D. T. R., & Nelson, N. W. (2010). DSM-5 and malingering: A modest proposal. *Psychological Injury & Law, 3*(4), 295–303.

Bieliauskas, L. A. (1999). Mediocrity is no standard: Searching for self-respect in clinical neuropsychology. *Clinical Neuropsychologist, 13*(1), 1–11.

Bilder, R. M. (2011). Neuropsychology 3.0: Evidence-Based Science and Practice. *Journal of the International Neuropsychological Society, 17*(1), 7–13.

Binder, L. M., & Kelly, M. P. (1996). Portland Digit Recognition Test performance by brain dysfunction patients without financial incentives. *Assessment, 3*(4), 403–409.

Boake, C. (2000). From Binet-Simon to the Wechsler-Bellevue: tracing the history of intelligence testing. *Journal of Clinical and Experimental Psychology, 24*(3), 383–405.

Boake, C. (2008). Clinical neuropsychology. *Professional Psychology: Research and Practice, 39*(2), 234–239.

Boake, C., Yeates, K. O., & Donders, J. (2002). Association of postdoctoral programs in clinical neuropsychology: Update and new directions. *The Clinical Neuropsychologist, 16*(1), 1–6.

Boone, K. B. (Ed.) (2007). *Assessment of feigned cognitive impairment: A neuropsychological perspective.* New York: Guilford Press.

Boone, K. B., Lu, P., & Wen, J. (2005). Comparison of various RAVLT scores in the detection of noncredible memory performance. *Archives of Clinical Neuropsychology, 20*(3), 301–320.

Boone, K. B., Lu, P., Back, C., King, C., Lee, A., Philpott, L., Shamieh, E., & Warner-Chacon, K. (2001). Sensitivity and specificity of the Rey Dot Counting Test in patients with suspect effort and various clinical samples. *Archives of Clinical Neuropsychology, 17*(7), 1–19.

Boone, K. B., Lu, P., Sherman, D., Palmer, B., Back, C., Shamieh, E., Warner-Chacon, K., & Berman, N. G. (2000). Validation of a new technique to detect malingering of cognitive symptoms: The b Test. *Archives of Clinical Neuropsychology, 15*(3), 227–241.

Boone, K. B., Salazar, X., Lu, P., Warner-Chacon, K., & Razani, J. (2002). The Rey 15-Item Recognition Trial: A technique to enhance sensitivity of the Rey 15-Item Memorization Test. *Journal of Clinical and Experimental Neuropsychology, 24*(5), 561–573.

Borg, J., Holm, L., Peloso, P. M., et al. (2004). Non-surgical intervention and cost for mild traumatic brain injury: results of the WHO Collaborating Centre Task Force on Mild Traumatic Brain Injury. *Journal of Rehabilitation Medicine, 43 (Supplement)*, 76–83.

Boring, E. G. (1950). *A history of experimental psychology*. New York: Appleton Century Crofts.

Brandt, J. & Benedict, R. H. B. (2001). *Hopkins Verbal Learning Test–Revised*. Odessa, FL: Psychological Assessment Resources.

Brickman, A. M., Cabo, R., & Manly, J. J. (2006). Ethical issues in cross-cultural neuropsychology. *Applied Neuropsychology, 13*(2), 91–100.

Brink, T. L., Yesavage, J. A., Lum, O., Heersema, P. H., Adey, M., & Rose, T. S. (1982). Screening tests for geriatric depression. *Clinical Gerontologist, 1*(1), 37–43.

Bulmer, M. G. (2003). *Francis Galton: pioneer of heredity and biometry*. Baltimore, MD: The Johns Hopkins University Press.

Bush, S. S. (2007). *Ethical decision making in clinical neuropsychology*. New York: Oxford University Press.

Bush, S. S. (2010). Determining whether or when to adopt new versions of psychological and neuropsychological tests: Ethical and professional considerations. *The Clinical Neuropsychologist, 24*(1), 7–16.

Bush, S. S., & Martin, T. A. (2006). Applied neuropsychology: Special issue ethical controversies in neuropsychology. *Applied Neuropsychology, 13*(2), 63–67.

Bush, S. S., Grote, C. L., Johnson-Greene, D. E., & Macartney-Filgate, M. (2008). A panel interview on the ethical practice of neuropsychology. *The Clinical Neuropsychologist, 22*(2), 321–344.

Butcher, J. N., Dahlstrom, W. G., Graham, J. R., Tellegen, A. M., & Kaemmer, B. (1989). *MMPI-2, Minnesota Multiphasic Personality Inventory–2: Manual for administration and scoring*. Minneapolis: University of Minnesota Press.

Butler, M., Retzlaff, P., & Vanderploeg, R. (1991). Neuropsychological test usage. *Professional Psychology: Research and Practice, 22*(6), 510–512.

Camara, W. J., Nathan, J. S., & Puente, A. E. (2000). Psychological test usage: Implications in professional psychology. *Professional Psychology: Research and Practice, 31*(2), 141–154.

Carone, D. A., Iverson, G. L., & Bush, S. S. (2010). A model to approaching and providing feedback to patients regarding invalid test performance in clinical neuropsychological evaluations. *The Clinical Neuropsychologist, 24*(5), 759–778.

Derouesne, C., Lacomblez, L., Thibault, S., & LePoncin, M. (1999). Memory complaints in young and elderly subjects. *International Journal of Geriatric Psychiatry, 14*(4), 291–301.

Chard, K. M., Schumm, J. A., Owens, G. P., & Cottingham, S. M. (2010). A comparison of OEF and OIF veterans and Vietnam veterans receiving cognitive processing therapy. *Journal of Traumatic Stress, 23*(1), 25–32.

Chelune, G. J. (2010). Evidence-based research and practice in clinical neuropsychology. *The Clinical Neuropsychologist, 24*(3), 454–467.

Christensen, A. L. (1975). *Luria's neuropsychological investigation.* New York: Spectrum.

Cicerone, K. D., Dahlberg, C., Kalmar, K., Langenbahn, K. M., Malec, J. F., Berquist, . . . Morse, P. A. (2000). Evidence-based cognitive rehabilitation: recommendations for clinical practice. *Archives of Physical Medicine and Rehabilitation, 81*(12), 1596–1615.

Cicerone, K. D., Dahlberg, C., Malec, J. F., Langenbahn, D. M., Felicetti, T., Kneipp, S., . . . Catanese, J. (2005). Evidence-based cognitive rehabilitation: Updated review of the literature from 1998 through 2002. *Archives Physical Medicine and Rehabilitation, 86*(8), 1681–1692.

Cohen, M. J. (1997). *Children's Memory Scale.* San Antonio, TX: The Psychological Corporation.

Conners, C. K., & MHS Staff. (2000). *Conners' Continuous Performance Test (CPT II) computer programs for Windows technical guide and software manual.* North Tonawanda, NY: Multi-Health Systems, Inc.

Costa, L. (1976). Clinical neuropsychology: Respice, adspice, and prospice. *The INS Bulletin,* 1–9.

Costa, L. (1998). Professional of neuropsychology: The early years. *The Clinical Neuropsychologist, 12*(1), 1–7.

Cox, D. R. (2010). Board certification in professional psychology: Promoting competency and consumer protection. *The Clinical Neuropsychologist, 24*(3), 493–505.

Crosson, B. (2000). Application of neuropsychological assessment results. In R. D. Vanderploeg (Ed.), *Clinician's guide to neuropsychological assessment* (2nd ed., pp. 195–244). Mahwah, NJ: Lawrence Erlbaum.

Delis, D. C., Kaplan, E. & Kramer, J. H. (2001). *Delis-Kaplan Executive Function System.* San Antonio, TX: The Psychological Corporation.

Delis, D. C., Kramer, J. H., Kaplan, E., & Ober, B. A. (2000). *California Verbal Learning Test-2nd Edition.* Adult version. San Antonio, TX: Psychological Corporation.

Demakis, G. J. (1999). Serial malingering on verbal and nonverbal fluency and memory measures: An analogue investigation. *Archives of Clinical Neuropsychology, 14*(4), 401–410.

Derouesne et al., (1999). Memory complaints in young and elderly subjects. *International Journal of Geriatric Psychiatry, 14*(4), 291–301.

Division 40, (1989). Definition of a clinical neuropsychologist. *The Clinical Neuropsychologist, 3*(1), 22.

Division 40, (2004). Official Position of the Division of Clinical Neuropsychology (APA Division 40) on the Role of Neuropsychologists in Clinical Use of fMRI: Approved by the Division 40 Executive Committee July 28, 2004,' *The Clinical Neuropsychologist, 18*(3), 349–351.

Donders, J. (2001a). A survey of report writing by neuropsychologists, I: General characteristics and content. *The Clinical Neuropsychologist, 15*(2), 137–149.

Donders, J. (2001b). A survey of report writing by neuropsychologists, II: Test data, report format, and document length. *The Clinical Neuropsychologist, 15*(2), 150–161.

Ernst, W. J., Pelletier, S. L., Simpson, G. (2008). Neuropsychological consultation with school personnel: what clinical neuropsychologists need to know. *The Clinical Neuropsychologist, 22*(6), 953–976.

Espiritu, Rashid, H., Mast, B. T., Fitzgerald, J., et al. (2001). Depression, cognitive impairment, and function in Alzheimer's disease. *International Journal of Geriatric Psychiatry, 16*(44), 1098–1103.

Fancher, R. E. (1998). Alfred Binet, general psychologist. In G. A. Kimble & M. Wertheimer (Eds.), *Portraits of pioneers in psychology*, (Vol 3). Washington, DC: American Psychological Association.

Faust, D., Hart, K., & Guilmette, T. (1988). Pediatric malingering: The capacity of children to fake believable deficits on neuropsychological testing. *Journal of Consulting and Clinical Psychology, 56*(4), 578–582.

Faust, D., Hart, K., Guilmette, T., & Arkes (1988). Neuropsychologist's capacity to detect adolescent malingering. *Professional Psychology: Research and Practice, 19*(5), 508–515.

Finger, S. (2001). *Origins of neuroscience: a history of explorations into brain function*. New York: Oxford University Press.

Finger, S. (2005). *Minds behind the brain: a history of the pioneers and their discoveries*. New York: Oxford University Press.

Finn, S. E., & Kamphuis, J. H. (2006). Therapeutic assessment with the MMPI-2. In J. N. Butcher (Ed.), *MMPI-2: A practitioner's guide* (pp. 165–191). Washington, DC: American Psychological Association.

Finn, S. E., & Tonsager, M. E. (1997). Information gathering and therapeutic models of assessment: Complementary paradigms. *Psychological Assessment, 9*(4), 374–338.

Fischer, C. T. (1994). *Individualizing psychological assessment*. Mahwah, NJ: Lawrence Erlbaum.

Fischer, C. T. (1994). Infusing humanistic perspectives into psychology. *Journal of Humanistic Psychology, 43*(3), 93–105.

Folstein, M. F., Folstein, S., & McHugh, P. R. (1975). "Mini-Mental State." A practical method for grading the cognitive state of patients for the clinician. *Journal of Psychiatric Research, 12*(3), 189–198.

Forsell, Y., & Winblad, B. (1998). Major depression in a population of demented and non-demented older people: Prevalence and correlates. *Journal of the American Geriatric Society, 46*(1), 27–30.

Franz, C. E., Barker, J. C., Kim, K., Flores, Y., Jenkins, C., Kravitz, R. L., Hinton, L. (2010). When help becomes a hindrance: mental health referral systems as barriers to care for primary care physicians treating patients with Alzheimer's disease. *American Journal of Geriatric Psychiatry, 18*(7), 576–585.

Galovski, T. E., & Resick, P. A. (2008). Cognitive processing therapy for posttraumatic stress disorder secondary to a motor vehicle accident: A single-subject report. *Cognitive and Behavioral Practice, 15*(4), 287–295.

Galski, T., Bruno, R. L., Zorowitz, R., & Walker, J. (1993). Predicting length of stay, functional outcome, and aftercare in the rehabilitation of stroke patients: The dominant role of higher-order cognition. *Stroke, 24*(12), 1794–1800.

Galton, F. (1879). Psychometric experiments. *Brain, 2*, 149–162.

Garrard, J., Rolnick, S.J., Nitz, N.M., Luepke, L., Jackson, J., Fischer, L. R., Leibson, C., Bland, P.C., Heinrich, R., & Waller, L. A. (1998). Clinical detection of depression among community-based elderly people with self-reported symptoms of depression. *Journals of Gerontology Series A: Biological Sciences and Medical Sciences, 53*(2), 92–101.

Gass, C. S., & Brown, M. C. (1992). Neuropsychological test feedback to patients with brain dysfunction. *Psychological Assessment, 4*(3), 272–277.

Gladsjo, J. A., Schuman, C. C., Evans, J. D., Peavy, G. M., Miller, S. W., & Heaton, R. K. (1999). Norms for letter and category fluency: Demographic corrections for age, education, and ethnicity. *Assessment, 6*(2), 147–178.

Golden, C. J. (1978). *Stroop Color and Word Test: A manual for clinical experimental uses.* Chicago: Stoelting Co.

Golden, C., Hammeke, T., & Purisch, A. (1978). Diagnostic validity of a standardized neuropsychological battery derived from Luria's neuropsychological tests. *Journal of Consulting and Clinical Psychology, 46*(6), 1258–1265.

Goldstein, G. (1990). Contributions of Kurt Goldstein to neuropsychology, *The Clinical Neuropsychologist, 4*(1), 3–17.

Goldstein, G., & Incagnoli, T., (Eds.). (1997). *Contemporary Approaches to Neuropsychological Assessment (Critical Issues in Neuropsychology).* New York: Plenum Press.

Goldstein, K., & Scheerer, M. (1941). Abstract and Concrete Behavior: An Experimental Study With Special Tests. *Psychological Monographs, 53*(2), 1–151.

GonzalezRothi, L. J., & Barrett, A. M. (2006). The changing view of neurorehabilitiation: a new era of optimism. *Journal of the International Neuropsychological Society, 12*(6), 812–815.

Goodglass, H., Kaplan, E., & Barresi, B. (2001). *Boston Diagnostic Aphasia Examination (3rd ed.).* Philadelphia: Lippincott Williams & Wilkins.

Goodglass, H., & Kaplan, E. (1979). Assessment of cognitive deficit in the brain-injured patient, In M. S. Gazzaniga (Ed.) *Handbook of behavioral neurology* (Vol. 2). New York: Plenum Press.

Gorske, T. T. & Smith, S. R. (2009). *Collaborative therapeutic neuropsychological assessment.* New York: Springer.

Grant, I., & Adams, K. M. (2009). *Neuropsychological assessment of neuropsychiatric and neuromedical disorders* (3rd Edition). New York: Oxford University Press.

Green, P. (2003). *Word Memory Test for Windows: User's manual and program.* Edmonton, Alberta, Canada: Author. (Revised 2005).

Green, P., & Iverson, G. L. (2001). Validation of the Computerized Assessment of Response Bias in litigating patients with head injuries. *The Clinical Neuropsychologist, 15*(4), 492–497.

Green, P., Rohling, M. L., Lees-Haley, P. R., & Allen, L. M. (2001). Effort has a greater effect on test scores than severe brain injury in compensation claimants. *Brain Injury, 15*(12), 1045–1060.

Greiffenstein, M. F., Baker, R., & Gola, T. (1994). Validation of malingered amnesia measures with a large clinical sample. *Psychological Assessment, 6*(3), 218–224.

Greiffenstein, M. F., Baker, W. J., & Gola, T. (1996). Motor dysfunction profiles in traumatic brain injury and postconcussion syndrome. *Journal of the International Neuropsychological Society, 2*(6), 477–485.

Gronwall, D. M. A. (1977). Paced Auditory Serial Addition Task: A measure of recovery from concussion. *Perceptual and Motor Skills, 44*(2), 367–373.

Guilmette, T. J., Hagan, L. D., & Giuliano, A. J. (2008). Assigning qualitative descriptions to test scores in neuropsychology: Forensic implications. *The Clinical Neuropsychologist, 22*(1), 122–139.

Gunstad, J., & Suhr, J. A. (2001). "Expectation as etiology" versus "the good old days": Postconcussion syndrome symptom reporting in athletes, headache sufferers, and depressed individuals. *Journal of the International Neuropsychological Society, 7*(3), 323–333.

Haaland, K. Y., Price, L., & Larue, A. (2003). What does the WMS-III tell us about memory changes with normal aging? *Journal of the International Neuropsychological Society, 9*(1), 89–96.

Halstead, W. (1947). *Brain and intelligence: A quantitative study of the frontal lobes.* Chicago: University of Chicago Press.

Hannay, H. J., Bieliauskas, L. A., Crosson, B. A., Hammeke, T. A., Hamsher, K. deS., & Koffler, S. P. (1998). Proceedings of the Houston conference on specialty education and training in clinical neuropsychology. *Archives of Clinical Neuropsychology, Special Issue, 13*(2), 157–250.

Heaton, R. K., Smith, H. H., Lehman, R. A. W., & Vogt, A. T. (1978). Prospects for faking believable deficits on neuropsychological testing. *Journal of Consulting and Clinical Psychology, 46*(5), 892–900.

Heaton, R. K., Chelune, G. J., Talley, J. L., Kay, G. G., & Curtis, G. (1993). *Wisconsin Card Sorting Test (WCST) Manual, revised and expanded.* Odessa, FL: Psychological Assessment Resources.

Heaton, R. K., Miller, S. W., Taylor, M. J., & Grant, I. (2004). *Revised comprehensive norms for an expanded Halstead-Reitan Battery: Demographically adjusted neuropsychological norms for African American and Caucasian adults.* Lutz, FL: Psychological Assessment Resources.

Heilbronner, R. L. (2007). American Academy of clinical neuropsychology (AACN) practice guidelines for neuropsychological assessment and consultation. *The Clinical Neuropsychologist, 21*(2), 209–231.

Heilbronner, R. L. (Ed.) (2008). *Neuropsychology in the courtroom: Expert analysis of reports and testimony.* New York: Guilford Press.

Heilbronner, R. L., Sweet, J. J., Morgan, J. E., Larrabee, G. J. Millis, S. R., & Conference Participants (2009). American Academy of Clinical Neuropsychology consensus conference statement on the neuropsychological assessment of effort, response bias, and malingering. *The Clinical Neuropsychologist, 23,* 1093–1129.

High, W. M., Sander, A. M., Struchen, M. A., & Hart, K. A. (Eds.). (2007). *Rehabilitation for traumatic brain injury.* New York: Oxford University Press.

Hooper, H. E. (1958). *The Hooper Visual Organization Test: Manual.* Beverly Hills, CA: Western Psychological Services.

Howe, L. L., Sweet, J. J., Bauer R. M. (2010). Advocacy 101: a step beyond complaining. How the individual practitioner can become involved and make a difference. *The Clinical Neuropsychologist, 24*(3), 373–390.

INS–Division 40 Task Force on Education, Accreditation, and Credentialing. (1987). Report of the INS–Division 40 Task Force on Education, Accreditation, and Credentialing. *Clinical Neuropsychologist, 1*(1), 29–34.

Ivnik, R. J., Malec, J. F., Smith, G. E., Tangalos, E. G., Peterson, R. C., Kokmen, E., & Kurland, L. T. (1992). Mayo's older American normative studies: WAIS-R, WMS-R and AVLT norms for ages 56 through 97. *The Clinical Neuropsychologist, 6*(Suppl.), 83–104.

Ivnik, R., Haaland, K., & Bieliauskas, L. A. (2000). The American Board of Clinical Neuropsychology (ABCN) 2000 update. *The Clinical Neuropsychologist, 14*(3), 261–268.

Jamora, C. W., Ruff, R. M., Connor, B. B. (2008). Geriatric neuropsychology: implications for front line clinicians. *NeuroRehabilitation, 23*(5), 381–394.

Johnson-Greene, D. (2005). Informed consent in clinical neuropsychology practice official statement of the National Academy of Neuropsychology. *Archives of Clinical Neuropsychology, 20*(3), 335–340.

Johnson-Greene, G., & Nissley, H. (2008). Ethical challenges in neuropsychology. In J. E. Morgan & J. H. Ricker (Eds.), *Textbook of Clinical Neuropsychology* (pp. 945–959). New York: Taylor & Francis.

Jurica, P. J., Leitten, C. L., & Mattis, S. (2001). *Dementia Rating Scale-2.* Odessa, FL: Psychologcial Assessment Resources.

Kanauss, K., Schatz, P., Puente, A. E. (2005). Current trends in the reimbursement of professional neuropsychological services. *Archives of Clinical Neuropsychology, 20*(3), 341–353.

Kaplan, E. F., Goodglass, H., & Weintraub, S. (2001). *The Boston Naming Test (2nd ed.).* Philadelphia: Lippincott Williams & Wilkins.

Kaplan, E., Fein, D., Morris, R., & Delis, D. C. (1991). WAIS-R as a Neuropsychological Instrument. San Antonio, TX: The Psychological Corporation.

Kaufmann, P. M. (2009). Protecting raw data and psychological tests from wrongful disclosure: A primer on the law and other persuasive strategies. *The Clinical Neuropsychologist, 23*(7), 1130–1159.

Kay, T. (1999). Interpreting apparent neuropsychological deficits: What is really wrong? In J.J. Sweet (Ed.), *Forensic neuropsychology: Fundamentals and practice* (pp. 145–183). Lisse, The Netherlands: Swets & Zeitlinger.

King, J.H., Sweet, J.J., Sherer, M., Curtiss, G., & Vanderploeg, R. (2002). Validity indicators within the Wisconsin Card Sorting Test: Application of new and previously researched multivariate procedures in multiple traumatic brain injury samples. *The Clinical Neuropsychologist, 16*(4), 506–523.

Klinkman, M., Coyne, J., Gallo, S., Schwenk, T. (1997). Can case finding instruments be used to improve physician detection of depression in primary care? *Archives of Family Medicine, 6*(6), 567–573.

Klonoff, P. S. (2010). *Psychotherapy after brain injury: Principles and techniques.* New York: Guilford Press.

Knopman, D. S., DeKosky, S. T., Cummings, J. L., Chui, H., Corey–Bloom, J., Relkin, . . . Stevens, J. C. (2001). Practice parameter: Diagnosis of dementia (an evidence-based review). Report of the Quality Standards Subcommittee of the American Academy of Neurology. *Neurology, 56*(9), 1143–1153.

Knox, H. (1914). A Scale, based on the Work at Ellis Island, for Estimating Mental Defect. *Journal of the American Medical Association, 62,* 741–747.

Korkman, M., Kirk, U., & Kemp, S. (1998). *NEPSY: A Developmental Neuropsychological Assessment manual.* San Antonio, TX: The Psychological Corporation.

Lamberty, G. J. (2002). Traditions and trends in clinical neuropsychology, in R. Ferraro (Ed.), *Minority and cross cultural aspects of neuropsychological assessment* (pp. 3–15). Lisse, The Netherlands: Swets & Zeitlinger.

Lamberty, G. J. (2007). *Understanding somatization in the practice of clinical neuropsychology.* New York: Oxford University Press.

Lamberty, G. J. (2009). President's annual state of the academy report. *The Clinical Neuropsychologist, 23*(1), 1–6.

Lamberty, G. J., Courtney, J. C., & Heilbronner, R. L. (Eds.) (2003). *The Practice of Clinical Neuropsychology*. Lisse, The Netherlands: Swets & Zeitlinger.

Larrabee, G. J. (2005). *Forensic neuropsychology: A scientific approach*. New York: Oxford University Press.

Larrabee, G. J., Millis, S. R., & Meyers, J. E. (2008). Sensitivity to brain dysfunction of the Halstead-Reitan vs. an ability-focused neuropsychological battery. *The Clinical Neuropsychologist, 22*(5), 813–825.

Leach, L., Kaplan, E., Rewilak, D., Richards, B., & Proulx G.-B. (2000). *Kaplan-Baycrest Neurocognitive Assessment (manual)*. San Antonio, TX: The Psychological Corporation.

Lezak, M. D. (2003). Principles of neuropsychological assessment. In T. E. Feinberg & M. J. Farah (Eds.) *Behavioral Neurology & Neuropsychology (2nd ed)*. New York, NY: McGraw-Hill.

Lezak, M. D., Howieson, D. B., Loring, D. W., Hannay, H. J., & Fischer, J. S. (2004). *Neuropsychological assessment* (4th ed.). New York: Oxford University Press.

Loring, D. W., & Larrabee, G. J. (2006). Sensitivity of the Halstead and Wechsler test batteries to brain damage: Evidence from Reitan's original validation sample. *The Clinical Neuropsychologist, 20*(2), 221–229.

Lu, P. Boone, K., B., Cozolino, L., & Mitchell, C. (2003). Effectiveness of the Rey-Osterrieth Complex Figure Test and the Meyers and Meyers recognition trial in the detection of suspect effort. *The Clinical Neuropsychologist, 17*(3), 426–440.

Lu, P., Boone, K. B., Jimenez, N., & Razani, J. (2004). Failure to inhibit the reading response on the Stroop Test: A pathognomonic indicator of suspect effort. *Journal of Clinical and Experimental Neuropsychology, 26*(2), 180–189.

Luria, A. R. (1966). *Human brain and psychological processes*. New York: Harper & Row.

Lysack, C. L., Neufeld, S., Mast, B. T., MacNeill, S. E., & Lichtenberg, P.A. (2003). After rehabilitation: An 18-month follow-up of elderly inner-city women. *American Journal of Occupational Therapy, 57*(3), 298–306.

Martin, T. A., & Bush, S. S. (2008). Ethical considerations in geriatric neuropsychology. *NeuroRehabilitation, 23*(5), 447–454.

McCaffrey, R. J., Palav, A. A., O'Bryant, S. E., & Labarge, A. S. (Eds.)(2003). *Practitioner's guide to symptom base rates in clinical neuropsychology*. New York: Kluwer Academic/ Plenum.

McCrea, M. (2007). *Mild traumatic brain injury and post-concussion syndrome: The New evidence base for diagnosis and treatment*. New York: Oxford University Press.

McCrea, M., Pliskin, N., Barth, J., Cox, D., Fink, J., French, L., . . . Yoash-Gantz, R. (2008). Official position of the military TBI task force on the role of neuropsychology and rehabilitation psychology in the evaluation, management, and research of military veterans with traumatic brain injury. *The Clinical Neuropsychologist, 22*(1), 10–26.

McGrew, K. S. (1997). Analysis of the major intelligence batteries according to a proposed comprehensive *Gf-Gc* framework. In D. P. Flanagan, J. L. Genshaft, & P. L. Harrison (Eds.), *Contemporary intellectual assessment: Theories, tests, and issues* (pp. 151–180). New York: Guilford.

McGrew, K. S., & Woodcock, R. W. (2001). *Woodcock-Johnson III technical manual*. Itasca, IL: Riverside Publishing.

Meier, M. J. (1992). Modem clinical neuropsychology in historical perspective. *American Psychologist, 47*(2), 550–558.

Meyer, G. J., Finn, S. E., Eyde, L. D., Kay, G. G., Moreland, K. L., Dies, R. R., . . . Read, G. M. (2001). Psychological testing and psychological assessment: A review of evidence and issues. *American Psychologist, 56*(2), 128–165.

Meyers, J. & Meyers, K. (1995). *The Meyers Scoring System for the Rey Complex Figure and the Recognition Trial: Professional manual.* Odessa, FL: Psychological Assessment Resources.

Milberg, W. P., Hebben, N., & Kaplan, E. (2009). The Boston Process Approach to neuropsychological assessment, In I. Grant & K. M. Adams (Eds.), *Neuropsychological assessment of neuropsychiatric and neuromedical disorders.* (pp. 42–65). New York: Oxford University Press.

Miller, L. S., & Rohling, M. L. (2001). A statistical interpretative method for neuropsychological test data. *Neuropsychology Review, 11*(3), 143–169.

Millis, S. R. (2004). Evaluation of Malingered Neurocognitive Disorders. In M. Rizzo & P. J. Eslinger (Eds.), *Principles and Practice of Behavioral Neurology and Neuropsychology.* Philadelphia, PA: Saunders.

Mindt, M. R., Byrd, D., Saez, P., & Manly, J. (2010). Increasing culturally competent neuropsychological services for ethnic minority populations: A call to action. *The Clinical Neuropsychologist, 24*(3), 429–453.

Mitrushina, M., Boone, K. B., Razani, J., & D'Elia, L. F. (2005). *Handbook of normative data for neuropsychological assessment* (2nd edition). Oxford: Oxford University Press.

Mittenberg, W., Canyock, E. M., Condit, D., & Patton, C. (2001). Treatment of post-concussion syndrome following mild head injury. *Journal of Clinical and Experimental Neuropsychology, 23*(6), 829–836.

Mittenberg, W., Theroux, S., Aguila-Puentes, G., Bianchini, K., Greve, K., & Rayls, K. (2001b). Identification of malingered head injury on the Wechsler Adult Intelligence Scale-3rd Edition. *The Clinical Neuropsychologist, 15*(4), 440–445.

Moberg, P. J., & Kniele, K. (2006). Evaluation of competency: Ethical considerations for neuropsychologists. *Applied Neuropsychology, 13*(2), 101–114.

Morey, L. C. (1991). *The Personality Assessment Inventory.* Odessa, FL: Psychological Assessment Inventory.

Morgan, J. E., & Ricker, J. H. (Eds.). (2008). *Textbook of clinical neuropsychology. Studies on neuropsychology, neurology and cognition.* New York, NY: Psychology Press.

National Academy of Neuropsychology. (2001). Definition of a clinical neuropsychologist. *Archives of Clinical Neuropsychology, 18*(5), 551–555.

Nelson, N. W., & Pontón, M. O. (2007). The art of clinical neuropsychology. In B. P. Uzzell, M. Pontón, & A. Ardila (Eds.), *International handbook of cross- cultural neuropsychology.* Mahway, NJ: Lawrence Erlbaum.

Nitch, S. Boone, K. B., Wen, J., Arnold, G., & Alfano, K. (2006). The utility of the Rey Word Recognition Test in the detection of suspect effort. *The Clinical Neuropsychologist, 20*(4), 873–887.

Olafsdottir, M., Skoog, I., Marcussion, J. (2000). Detection of dementia in primary care: the Linkoping study. *Dementia and Geriatric Cognitive Disorders, 11*(4), 223–229.

Otto, M. W., Bruder, G. E., Fava, M., Delis, D. C., Quitkin, F. M., & Rosenbaum, J. F. (1994). Norms for depressed patients for the California Verbal Learning Test: Associations with depression severity and self-report of cognitive difficulties. *Archives of Clinical Neuropsychology, 9*(1), 81–88.

Ownby, R. L. (1990). A study of the expository process model in school psychological reports. *Psychology in the Schools, 27*(4), 353–358.

Ownby, R. L. (1997). *Psychological reports: A guide to report writing in professional psychology* (3rd edition). New York: John Wiley.

Paige, R. U., & Robinson, E. A. (2003). The prescriptive authority agenda: Evolving structures and efforts in the American Psychological Association. In M. T. Sammons, R. U. Paige, & R. F. Levant (Eds.), *Prescriptive authority for psychologists: A history and guide* (pp. 59–75). American Psychological Association, Washington DC.

Palmer, B. W., Boone, K. B., Lessler, I. M., & Wohl, M. A. (1998). Base rates of "impaired" neuropsychological test performance among healthy older adults. *Archives of Clinical Neuropsychology, 13*(6), 503–511.

Pankratz, L., Fausti, S. A., & Peed, S. (1975). A forced-choice technique to evaluate deafness in the hysterical or malingering patient. *Journal of Consulting and Clinical Psychology, 43*(3), 421–422.

Petersen, R.C., Stevens, J.C., Ganguli, M., Tangalos, E. G., Cummings, J. L., & DeKosky, S. T. (2001). Practice parameter: Early detection of dementia: Mild cognitive impairment (an evidence-based review). Report of the Quality Standards Subcommittee of the American Academy of Neurology. *Neurology, 56*(9), 1133–1142.

Porter, T. M. (2004). *Karl Pearson: the scientific life in a statistical age*. Princeton, NJ: Princeton University Press.

Prigatano, G. (1999). *Principles of neuropsychological rehabilitation*. New York: Oxford University Press.

Prigatano, G. P. (2008). Neuropsychological rehabilitation and psychodynamic psychotherapy. In J. E. Morgan, & J. H. Ricker (Eds.), (pp. 985–995). New York: Psychology Press.

Puente, A. E., & Marcotte, A. C. (2000). A history of Division 40 (Clinical Neuropsychology). In D. A. Dewsbury (Ed.), *Unification through division: Histories of the divisions of the American Psychological Association, vol. V.* (pp. 137–160). Washington, DC: American Psychological Association.

Putnam, S. H. (1989). The TCN salary survey: A salary survey of neuropsychologists. *Clinical Neuropsychologist, 3*(2), 97–115.

Rabin, L. A., Barr, W. B., & Burton, L. A. (2005). Assessment practices of clinical neuropsychologists in the United States and Canada: A survey of INS, NAN, and APA Division 40 members. *Archives of* Clinical Neuropsychology, *20*(1), 33–65.

Randolph, C. (1998). *RBANS manual*. San Antonio, TX: The Psychological Corporation.

Reger, M. A., Welsh, R. K., Watson, G. S., Cholerton, B., Baker, L. D., & Craft, S. (2004). The relationship between neuropsychological functioning and driving ability in dementia: A meta-analysis. *Neuropsychology, 18*(1), 85–93.

Reitan, R. M. (1955). The relation of the Trail Making Test to organic brain damage. *Journal of Consulting Psychology, 19*(5), 393–394.

Reitan, R. M. (1994). Ward Halstead's contributions to neuropsychology and the Halstead-Reitan Neuropsychological Test Battery. *Journal of Clinical Psychology, 50*(1), 47–70.

Reitan, R. M., & Wolfson, D. (1985). *The Halstead-Reitan neuropsychological test battery: Theory and clinical interpretation*. Tucson, AZ: Neuropsychology Press.

Reitan, R. M., & Wolfson, D. (1995). Category Test and Trail Making Test as measures of frontal lobe functions. *The Clinical Neuropsychologist, 9*(1), 50–56.

Reitan, R. M., & Wolfson, D. (2009). The Halstead Reitan Neuropsychological Test Battery for adults – theoretical, methodological, and validational bases. In I. Grant & K. M. Adams (Eds.), *Neuropsychological assessment of neuropsychiatric and neuromedical disorders.* (pp. 3–24). New York: Oxford University Press.

Reitan, R. M., Hom, J., Van De Voorde, J., Stanczak, D. E., Wolfson, D. (2004). The Houston Conference revisited. *Archives of Clinical Neuropsychology, 19*(3), 375–390.

Reports of the INS-Division 40 Task Force on Education, Accreditation, and Credentialing (1987). *The Clinical Neuropsychologist, 1*(1), 29–34.

Reynolds, C. R. (2002). An essay on the Houston conference policy statement: Static yet incomplete or a work in progress? *Neuropsychology Review, 12*(3), 143–145.

Robinson, P. J. (2009). From behavioral analysis to insight: Using ACT to advance psychotherapy. *PsycCRITIQUES, 54*(34).

Rohling, M. L., Lees-Haley, P. R., Langhinrichsen-Rohling, J., & Williamson, D. J. (2003). A statistical analysis of board certification in clinical neuropsychology. *Archives of Clinical Neuropsychology, 18*(4), 331–352.

Rohling, M. L., Williamson, D. J., Miller, L. S., & Adams, R. L. (2003). Using the Halstead-Reitan battery to diagnose brain damage: A comparison of the predictive power of traditional techniques to Rohling's interpretive method. *The Clinical Neuropsychologist, 17*(4), 531–543.

Roid, G. H. (2003). *Stanford-Binet Intelligence Scales, Fifth Edition.* Itasca, IL: Riverside Publishing.

Rollnick, S., Miller, W. R., & Butler, C. C. (2008). *Motivational interviewing in health care: Helping patients change behavior.* New York: Guilford.

Romero, H. R., Lageman, S. K., Kamath, V., Irani, F., Sim, A., et al. (2009). Challenges in the neuropsychological assessment of ethnic minorities: Summit proceedings. *The Clinical Neuropsychologist, 23*(5), 761–779.

Rourke, B. P. & Murji, S. (2000). A history of the international neuropsychological society: The early years (1965–1985). *Journal of the International Neuropsychological Society, 6*(4), 491–509.

Royall, D. R., Cordes, J. a., & Polk, M. (1998). CLOX: an executive clock drawing task. *Journal of Neurology, Neurosurgery, & Psychiatry, 64*(5), 588–594.

Ruchinskas, (2002). Rehabilitation therapists' recognition of cognitive and mood disorders in geriatric patients. *Archives of Physical Medicine & Rehabilitation, 83*(5), 609–612.

Ruff, R. (1996, 1998). *Ruff Figural Fluency Test.* Odessa, FL: Psychological Assessment Resources.

Ruff, R. (2003). A friendly critique of neuropsychology: Facing the challenges of our future. *Archives of Clinical Neuropsychology, 18*(8), 847–864.

Russell, E. W. (1997). Developments in the psychometric foundations of neuropsychological assessment. In G. Goldstein, & T. M. Incagnoli (Eds.), *Contemporary Approaches to Neuropsychological Assessment* (pp. 15–65). New York: Plenum Press.

Russell, E. W. (2009). Commentary on Larrabee, Millis, and Meyers' paper "sensitivity to brain dysfunction of the Hallstead Reitan vs. an ability-focused neuropsychological battery." *The Clinical Neuropsychologist, 23*(5), 831–840.

Sackett, D. L., Straus, S. E., Richardson, W. S., Rosenberg, W., & Haynes, R. B. (2000). *Evidence-based medicine: How to practice and teach EBM (2nd ed.).* New York: Churchill Livingston.

Sattler, J. M. (1992). *Assessment of children* (3rd edition). San Diego, CA: Sattler.

Schacter, D. L. (1986a). On the relation between genuine and simulated amnesia. *Behavioral Sciences and the Law, 4(1)*, 47–64.

Schacter, D. L. (1986b). Amnesia and crime: how much do we really know? *American Psychologist, 41(3)*, 286–295.

Schoenberg, M. R., Duff, K., Scott, J. G., & Adams, R. L. (2003). An evaluation of the clinical utility of the OPIE-3 as an estimate of premorbid WAIS-III FSIQ. *The Clinical Neuropsychologist, 17(3)*, 308–321.

Schoenberg, M. R., Scott, J. G., Duff, K., & Adams, R. L. (2002). Estimation of WAIS-III intelligence from combined performance and demographic variables: Development of the OPIE-3. *The Clinical Neuropsychologist, 16(4)*, 426–438.

Schretlen, D. (1997). *Brief Test of Attention professional manual*. Odessa, FL: Psychological Assessment Resources.

Schretlen, D. J., Munro, C. A., Anthony, J. C., & Pearlson, G. D. (2003). Examining the range of normal intraindividual variability in neuropsychological test performance. *Journal of the International Neuropsychological Society, 9(6)*, 864–870.

Schretlen, D. J., Testa, S. M., Winicki, J. M., Pearlson, G. D., & Gordon, B. (2008). Frequency and bases of abnormal performance by healthy adults on neuropsychological testing. *Journal of the International Neuropsychological Society, 14(3)*, 436–445.

Siegler, R. S. (1992). The other Alfred Binet. *Developmental Psychology, 28(2)*, 179–190.

Slick, D. J. Hopp, G. Strauss, E., & Spellacy, F. J. (1996). Victoria Symptom Validity Test: Efficiency for detecting feigned memory impairment and relationship to neuropsychological tests and MMPI-2 validity scales. *Journal of Clinical and Experimental Neuropsychology, 18(6)*, 911–922.

Slick, D. J., Sherman, E. M. S., & Iverson, G. L. (1999). Diagnostic criteria for malingered neurocognitive dysfunction: Proposed standards for clinical practice and research. *The Clinical Neuropsychologist, 13(4)*, 545–561.

Smith, G. E., Ivnik, R. J., & Lucas, J. (2008). Assessment techniques: Tests, test batteries, norms and methodological approaches. In J. E. Morgan & J. H. Ricker (Eds.), *Textbook of Clinical Neuropsychology* (pp. 38–57). New York: Taylor & Francis.

Smith-Seemiller, L., Franzen, M. D., Burgess, E. J., & Prieto, L. R. (1997). Neuropsychologists' practice patterns in assessing premorbid intelligence. *Archives of Clinical Neuropsychology, 12(8)*, 739–744.

Sohlberg, M. M., & Mateer, C. A. (2001). *Cognitive rehabilitation: An Integrative neuropsychological approach*. New York: Guilford.

Sternberg, R.J., & Grigorenko, E.L. (1997). *Intelligence, heredity, and environment*. New York: Cambridge University Press.

Stevens, R. (1978). *American medicine in the public interest*. New Haven, CT: Yale University Press.

Strauss, E., Sherman, E. M. S., & Spreen, O. (2006). *A compendium of neuropsychological tests: Administration, norms, and commentary* (2nd ed.). New York: Oxford University Press.

Stucky, K. J., Bush, S., & Donders, J. (2010). Providing effective supervision in clinical neuropsychology. *The Clinical Neuropsychologist, 24(5)*, 737–758.

Suchy, Y., & Sweet, J. J. (2000). Information/Orientation subtest of the Wechsler Memory Scale-Revised as an indicator of suspicion of insufficient effort. *The Clinical Neuropsychologist, 14(1)*, 56–66.

Sweet, J. J. & Moberg, P. (1990). A survey of practices and beliefs among ABPP and non-ABPP clinical neuropsychologists. *The Clinical Neuropsychologist, 4*(2), 101–120.

Sweet, J. J. (1999). *Forensic Neuropsychology: Fundamentals and practice.* Lisse, The Netherlands: Swets and Zeitlinger.

Sweet, J. J. (2008). President's annual state of the Academy report. *The Clinical Neuropsychologist, 22*(1), 1–9.

Sweet, J. J. & King, J. H. (2002). Category Test validity indicators: Overview and practice recommendations. *Journal of Forensic Neuropsychology, 3*(1–2), 241–274.

Sweet, J. J., King, J. H., Malina, A. C., Bergman, M. A., & Simmons, A. (2002). Documenting the prominence of forensic neuropsychology at national meetings and in relevant professional journals from 1990 to 2000. *The Clinical Neuropsychologist, 16*(4), 481–494.

Sweet, J.J., Giuffre Meyer, D. Nelson, N.W., & Moberg, P. (2011). The TCN/AACN "Salary Survey": Professional practices, beliefs, and incomes of U.S. neuropsychologists. *The Clinical Neuropsychologist, 25*(1), 12–61.

Sweet, J. J., Moberg, P., & Suchy, Y. (2000). Ten-year follow-up survey of clinical neuropsychologists: Part I. Practices and beliefs. *The Clinical Neuropsychologist, 14*(1), 18–37.

Sweet, J. J., Nelson, N. W., & Moberg, P. J. (2006). The TCN/AACN 2005 "salary survey": Professional practices, beliefs and incomes of U. S. neuropsychologists. *The Clinical Neuropsychologist, 20*(3), 325–364.

Sweet, J. J., Westergaard, C. J., & Moberg, P. J. (1995). "Managed care experiences of clinical neuropsychologists, *The Clinical Neuropsychologist, 9*(3), 214–218.

Sweet, J. J., Wolfe, P., Sattlberger, E., Neuman, B., Rosenfeld, J.P., Clingerman, S., & Nies, K.J. (2000). Further investigation of traumatic brain injury versus insufficient effort with the California Verbal Learning Test. *Archives of Clinical Neuropsychology, 15*(2), 105–113.

The Psychological Corporation (1997). *WAIS-III-WMS-III technical manual.* San Antonio, TX: Author.

The Psychological Corporation (2002). *Wechsler Individual Achievement Test–2nd Edition.* San Antonio, TX: Author.

Tombaugh, T. N. (1996). *Test of Memory Malingering.* Toronto, ON: Multi Health Systems.

Tranel, D. (2009). The Iowa-Benton School of neuropsychological assessment. In I. Grant & K. M. Adams (Eds.), *Neuropsychological assessment of neuropsychiatric and neuromedical disorders.* (pp. 66–83). New York: Oxford University Press.

Van Hout, H., Vernooij-Dassen, M., Poels, P., Hoefnagels, W., Grol, R. (2000). Are general practitioners able to accurately diagnoses dementia and identify Alzheimer's disease? A comparison with an outpatient memory clinic. *British Journal of General Practice, 50*(453), 311–312.

Vanderploeg, R. D. (2000). *Clinician's guide to neuropsychological assessment.* Mahwah, NJ: Lawrence Erlbaum.

Wachtel, P. L. (2010). Beyond "ESTs": Problematic assumptions in the pursuit of evidence-based practice. *Psychoanalytic Psychology, 27*(3), 251–272.

Wechsler, D. (1991). *Wechsler Intelligence Scale for Children-Third Edition.* San Antonio, TX: Psychological Corporation.

Wechsler, D. (1997). *Wechsler Adult Intelligence Scale-Third Edition.* San Antonio, TX: Psychological Corporation.

Wechsler, D. (2003). *Wechsler Intelligence Scale for Children-Fourth Edition.* San Antonio, TX: Psychological Corporation.

Wechsler, D. (2008). *Wechsler Adult Intelligence Scale-Fourth Edition*. San Antonio, TX: Pearson.

Wilkinson, G. S., & Robertson, G. J. (2006). *WRAT4 Wide Range Achievement Test professional manual (4th ed.)*. Lutz, FL: Psychological Assessment Resources.

Wilson, B. A., & Glisky, E. L. (2009). *Memory Rehabilitation: Integrating theory and practice*. New York: Guilford.

Yeates, K. O. & Bieliauskas, L. A. (2004). The American Board of Clinical Neuropsychology and the American Academy of Clinical Neuropsychology: Milestones past and present. *The Clinical Neuropsychologist, 18*(4), 489–493.

Yeates, K. O. Ris, D. M., Taylor, H. G., Pennington, B. F., (Eds.). (2010). *Pediatric neuropsychology: Research, theory and practice (2nd Ed.)*. New York: Guilford Press.

Yerkes, R.M. (Ed.) (1921). Psychological examining in the United States Army. *Memoirs of the National Academy of Sciences, 15* (Parts 1–3), Washington, DC: Government Printing Office.

Zigler, E. & Gilman, E. (1998). The legacy of Jean Piaget. In G. A. Kimble & M. Wertheimer (Eds.), *Portraits of pioneers in psychology*, (Vol 3). Washington, DC: American Psychological Association.

Zimmer, (2004). *Soul made flesh: The discovery of the brain and how it changed the world*. New York: Free Press.

KEY TERMS

Boston Process approach—an assessment approach that focuses on qualitative aspects of behaviors observed in the clinical neuropsychological exam, and relating this information to a broader theoretical understanding of cognition.

Case Conceptualization—a process that incorporates assessment findings with additional forms of information to assist the clinician's understanding of the patient's level of function.

Clinical Neuropsychology Synarchy (CNS)—a collective of organizations involved in clinical neuropsychology education, training, and practice advocacy which has as its goal a unified approach to issues confronting the neuropsychology practice community.

Commission for the Recognition of Specialties and Proficiencies in Professional Psychology (CRSPPP)—a commission from within APA that is responsible for reviewing petitions from organizations requesting the association's recognition of a professional specialty or proficiency.

Factor analysis—a method of statistical analysis that examines the interrelationships among a set of continuously measured variables by a number of underlying, linearly independent reference variables called factors. Factor analysis has been important in psychological and neuropsychological measurement contexts.

Flexible battery approach—an assessment approach that utilizes a core set of measures to assess neuropsychological functioning and augments that core set of measures with additional tests as dictated by the clinical facts of a case.

Functionalist approach—an approach in early American psychology that emphasized the organism's adaptation to the environment, rather than a specific focus on structure and individual experience as was common in the first laboratories of psychology.

Gestalt approach—an approach in early psychology that stressed phenomenological observation and appreciation of the whole as opposed to individual parts. This also involved more emphasis on dynamics or processes in understanding overall functioning.

Halstead–Reitan Neuropsychological Test Battery (HRB)—a battery of specific neuropsychological tasks, many of which were originally developed and used by W. Halstead in his work *Biological Intelligence*. These measures were subsequently augmented and normed by Halstead's student, R. Reitan. The HRB was arguably the driving force behind a scientifically oriented clinical neuropsychology.

Houston Conference—a meeting in September of 1997 of 37 individuals broadly involved in education, training, and practice in clinical neuropsychology, whose aim was to "advance an aspirational, integrated model of specialty training in clinical neuropsychology." The HC model is now the standard of training for those seeking board certification in clinical neuropsychology through the American Board of Clinical Neuropsychology.

Idiographic knowledge—knowledge that is derived from the study of individual behavior with aim toward how he or she is unique or distinct from others. In clinical neuropsychology, idiographic knowledge is derived from exploration of the individual's *subjective* experience of cognition, emotion, and behavior. Idiographic knowledge is typically integrated with nomothetic ("lawful") knowledge to inform a holistic understanding of the individual.

Independent Medical Evaluation (IME)—An examination process that entails comprehensive assessment of an individual's physical, cognitive, psychological, and/or behavioral functioning, usually conducted on behalf of an individual's insurance company or employer to ascertain whether claimed difficulties render an individual disabled. Unlike clinical evaluation settings, in which the neuropsychologist is working on behalf of the individual (as a treater or patient advocate), the role of the neuropsychologist in an IME setting is as an expert who is requested to offer an opinion regarding functional status independent of how this may impact the individual's clinical care.

Intelligence Quotient (IQ)—a simple index, originally proposed by W. Stern, to characterize general intellectual ability as a function of demonstrated abilities and chronological age (mental age/chronological age). L. Terman would later multiply this term by 100 to get the familiar IQ score.

Nomothetic knowledge—knowledge that is derived from "lawful" explanations of human behavior through the study of large groups. In clinical neuropsychology, nomothetic knowledge is derived from the study of specific variables that impact *objective* cognitive performances in large normative groups. Significant deviations from normative distributions of performance suggest "impairment" or cognitive dysfunction. Nomothetic knowledge is typically integrated with idiographic (individual-specific) knowledge to inform a holistic understanding of the individual.

Performance tests—also known as ability tests, performance tests are neuropsychological measures developed with the specific intent to assess a specific cognitive ability or capacity. Common areas of performance in clinical neuropsychology include attention/concentration, language, visual-spatial, executive, and learning/memory function. Individual performances are usually compared against normative benchmarks from large normative samples to identify levels of function, from impaired to superior.

Probability distributions—in mathematics, a function that describes the probability of a random variable taking certain values. In neuropsychology, continuous probability distributions are used to describe the likelihood of performances on specific tests, which allow characterization of scores in terms of clinical impairment. This typically involves the assumption of a normal distribution.

Psychometrics—a domain of study devoted to the formal assessment of a theoretical psychological or cognitive construct. Psychometrics in clinical neuropsychology pertain to the development and study of a wide array of instruments devoted to the formal evaluation of cognitive and behavioral functioning.

Symptom Validity Testing (SVT)—a procedure of assessing the reliability or legitimacy of an individual's cognitive performance on formal neuropsychological evaluation. SVT instruments are developed with the sole purpose of identifying whether issues of insufficient effort, diminished task engagement, or intentional subversion of performance render a neuropsychological profile invalid or uninterpretable.

AACN. *See* American Academy of Clinical
Neuropsychology
AACN Foundation (AACNF), 25
AACN Practice Guidelines for
Neuropsychological Assessment and
Consultation
background of guideline development
process, 166–67
definitions, 146–47
education and training, 147–48
ethical and clinical issues, 149–52
introduction, 144–46
methods and procedures, 152–61
outline, 146
purpose and scope, 147
work settings, 148–49
ABCN. *See* American Board of Clinical
Neuropsychology
Ability tests. *See* Performance tests
ABMS. *See* American Board of Medical
Specialties
ABPN. *See* American Board of Psychiatry
and Neurology
Academic achievement assessment, 40*t*
Academic history, in neuropsychological
evaluation report, 74–75
Accommodation, 7
Accreditation. *See also* INS/Division 40 Task
Force on Education, Accreditation, and
Credentialing
Division 40 work in, 15–19
INS work in, 15–16
Activities of daily living (ADLs), in
neuropsychological evaluation
report, 74
Administration, test, 157
Advocacy for clinical
neuropsychology, 118–21
Affect observation, 71
Affordable Care Act, 114
Alliances. *See* Professional alliances
Allied health, consultation with, 90–92, 91*t*

American Academy of Clinical
Neuropsychology (AACN), 24–26.
See also AACN Practice Guidelines for
Neuropsychological Assessment and
Consultation
ethics policy statements of, 99–100
outcomes research funded by, 122
on response validity assessment, 48
American Board of Clinical Neuropsychology
(ABCN)
board certification by, 23, 116–18, 116*f*,
117*f*, 145
credentialing and practice guidelines
of, 24–26
HC guideline use by, 20–21
American Board of Medical Specialties
(ABMS), 29
American Board of Psychiatry and Neurology
(ABPN), subspecialties of, 29–30
American Psychological Association
(APA), Division 40 of, 15–19,
22–23, 131
APA ethical guidelines/standards, 99,
145, 147
competence considerations in, 102–3
feedback considerations, 112
informed consent considerations, 103–5
referral question considerations in, 100
release of information
considerations, 110–12
report writing considerations, 109–10
test selection considerations, 105–9
APPCN. *See* Association of Postdoctoral
Programs in Clinical Neuropsychology
Army Alpha test, 8–9
Army Beta test, 8–9
Arousal, 55
Assessment, 33–35, 34*t*. *See also* Case
conceptualization; Cognitive
functioning assessment
AACN methods and procedures
for, 152–61

Assessment (*continued*)
  Boston Process approach to, 37–39
  as clinical neuropsychologist's role,
    26–27
  as clinical neuropsychology
    foundation, 9–12
  commonly employed instruments in, 43
  decision to go ahead with, 152
  of emotional functioning, 26–27, 55–57
  ethical considerations during, 103–10
  flexible battery approach to, 35–37, 39–40,
    40t–42t
  interpretation of, 157–59
  of personality, 56–57
  of response validity and effort, 42t, 46–51,
    55, 156
  skills needed for, 136–37
  standardized batteries for, 35–37, 36t
  test selection in, 51–53, 105–9, 151–52
  theoretical assumptions relevant to,
    53–55
  third-party, 149–51
  as unique evaluation process, 45–46
Assimilation, 7
Association of Postdoctoral Programs in
    Clinical Neuropsychology
    (APPCN), 96
Attention/concentration assessment, 40t–41t,
    54–55
Attorneys, consultation with, 92–94, 93t

Background. *See* Patient background
Base rates, 58–59
Batteries. *See also* Flexible battery approach
  fixed, 12, 34–35
  HRB, 10, 35–37, 36t, 183
  Luria Nebraska Neuropsychological
    Battery, 37
  standardized, 35–37, 36t
Beck Depression Inventory–2nd Edition
    (BDI-II), 57
Behavioral observations
  gait and movement, 70
  mood and affect, 71
  in neuropsychological evaluation
    report, 68–72
  presentation and demeanor, 69–70
  relationship to examiner, 71–72
  speech and language, 70–71
  task approach, 71–72
Benton, Arthur, 11–12
Benton approach. *See* Iowa-Benton School of
    Neuropsychological Assessment
Bieliauskas, Linas, 20
Binet, Alfred, 6–7

Binet–Simon scale, 7–8
Board certification, 18–23, 143
  ABCN, 23, 116–18, 116f, 117f, 145
  ABMS, 29
  competence and, 102–3
  future of, 115–18, 116f, 117f
Boston Process approach (BPA), 183
  as assessment strategy, 37–39
  in clinical neuropsychology
    foundations, 11
Brain injury
  educationally oriented intervention for, 95
  psychotherapy for individuals with, 89–90
Broca, Paul, 4
Buros Mental Measurement Yearbook, 43

California Verbal Learning Test-II, 38
Case conceptualization, 44–45
  base rates in, 58–59
  cognitive functioning assessment
    in, 51–55
  defined, 183
  demographic considerations in, 51–53
  emotional functioning and personality
    assessment in, 55–57
  population-based, 58–59
  pre-morbid background considerations
    in, 51–53
  response validity and effort assessment
    in, 42t, 46–51, 55
  test selection in, 51–53
  theoretical assumptions relevant to, 53–55
  unique process of, 45–46
CBT. *See* Cognitive behavioral therapy
Centers for Medicare and Medicaid Services
    (CMS), clinical neuropsychology
    advocacy and, 118–19
Certification. *See* Board certification
Charcot, Jean-Martin, 4–5, 10
Clinical medicine, in clinical
    neuropsychology foundations, 4–5
Clinical neuropsychology
  advocacy for, 118–21
  clinical medicine influences on, 4–5
  commonly employed instruments in, 43
  consumer's perspective of, 23–26
  as CRSPPP specialty area, 17–19
  defined, 3, 16–18, 21–23, 131–33, 135,
    142–43, 146–47
  dichotomies used in, 33–34, 34t
  Division 40 definition of, 16, 18, 22–23, 131
  Division 40 work in, 15–19
  EBPP and outcomes focus in, 121–23
  HC work in, 19–21
  historical background of, 3–12

historical milestones in, 14t
INS work in, 14–16
intelligence testing in, 6–9
NAN definition of, 21–23, 142–43
neuropsychological assessment
    foundations in, 9–12
populations served by, 27–29, 132
problems addressed by, 26–27, 26t
professional identity in, 115–18, 116f, 117f
psychometric influences on, 5–12
standardized batteries in, 35–37, 36t
subspecialization in, 29–30, 139
unique evaluation process in, 45–46
Clinical Neuropsychology Synarchy
    (CNS), 26, 183
Clinical referral sources, 90–92, 91t
CMS. *See* Centers for Medicare and
    Medicaid Services
CNS. *See* Clinical Neuropsychology Synarchy
Cognitive behavioral therapy (CBT), 89
Cognitive domains, 53–55
    measures categorized by, 40t–42t
Cognitive functioning assessment
    as clinical neuropsychologist's role, 26–27
    demographic considerations in, 51–53
    measures for, 40t–42t
    pre-morbid background considerations
        in, 51–53
    test selection in, 51–53
    theoretical assumptions relevant to, 53–55
Cognitive impairment
    psychotherapy for individuals with, 89–90
    subjective, 73–74
Cognitive rehabilitation, 87–89
Collaborative therapeutic neuropsychological
    assessment, 87
Collateral information, in neuropsychological
    evaluation report, 78
Commission for the Recognition of
    Specialties and Proficiencies in
    Professional Psychology (CRSPPP), 183
    clinical neuropsychology as specialty
        area of, 17–19
Competence, 102–3
Concentration. *See* Attention/concentration
    assessment
Conceptual foundations of clinical
    neuropsychology, 3
    clinical medicine influences, 4–5
    intelligence testing, 6–9
    neuropsychological assessment, 9–12
    psychometric influences, 5–12
Concurrent validity, 156–57
Confidentiality, 104
Consent. *See* Informed consent

Consultation. *See* Intervention and
    consultation
Consumer perspective, 23–26
Continuing education, 139
Costa, Louis, 15
Course of complaint, in neuropsychological
    evaluation report, 73–74
Credentialing. *See also* Board certification;
    INS/Division 40 Task Force on
    Education, Accreditation, and
    Credentialing
    ABCN and AACN work in, 24–26
    Division 40 work in, 15–19
    future of, 115–18, 116f, 117f
    INS work in, 15–16
Cross-cultural patients, 107–9, 151–52
CRSPPP. *See* Commission for the Recognition
    of Specialties and Proficiencies in
    Professional Psychology
Culture considerations, 107–9, 151–52

Demeanor, patient, 69–70
Demographic assessment
    considerations, 51–53
Depression, 55–57
Developmental psychology, in clinical
    neuropsychology foundations, 6–7
Diagnostic impressions, in
    neuropsychological evaluation
    report, 79–80
Disclosure, 104, 111–12
Diversity. *See also* Culture
    in education and training, 140
Division 40, 15–19. *See also* INS/Division 40
    Task Force on Education, Accreditation,
    and Credentialing
    clinical neuropsychology defined by, 16,
        18, 22–23, 131
Doctoral training programs
    HC policy statement on, 138
    INS/Division 40 Task Force on Education,
        Accreditation, and Credentialing
        guidelines for, 125–27

EBPP. *See* Evidence-based practice in
    psychology
Ecologic validity, 155
Education and training. *See also* Houston
    Conference; INS/Division 40 Task Force
    on Education, Accreditation, and
    Credentialing
    AACN practice guidelines for, 147–48
    diversity in, 140
    neuropsychologist role in, 94–95
    skills needed for, 137–38

Effort assessment, 42*t*, 46–51, 55, 156
Emotional functioning
    assessment of, 26–27, 55–57
    in neuropsychological evaluation
        report, 77–78
Ethical standards of practice, 99–100,
        145, 147
    AACN Practice Guidelines statement
        on, 149–52
    competence considerations, 102–3
    during evaluation phase, 103–10
    feedback considerations, 112
    informed consent considerations,
        103–5, 149
    during post-evaluation phase, 110–12
    during pre-evaluation phase, 100–103
    referral question considerations, 100–102
    release of information
        considerations, 110–12, 151
    report writing considerations, 109–10
    test selection considerations, 105–9,
        151–52
Ethnicity considerations, 107–9, 151–52
Evaluation. *See* Assessment
Evidence-based practice in psychology
        (EBPP), 23–24, 115, 121–23
Examiner, patient relationship with, 71–72
Executive functioning assessment, 41*t*, 54

Factitious disorders. *See* Malingering
Factor analysis, 6, 183
Familiar other
    interview of, 153–54
    in neuropsychological evaluation
        report, 78
Family consultation, 86–87
Family history, in neuropsychological
        evaluation report, 76
Feedback. *See* Patient feedback
Fellows, supervision of, 95–96
Ferrier, David, 4
Fixed battery approach, 12, 34–35
Flexible approach, 39–40
Flexible battery approach
    as assessment strategy, 35–37, 39–40,
        40*t*–42*t*
    in clinical neuropsychology
        foundations, 12
    defined, 183
    test selection for, 52
Forced-choice effort measures, 49–50
Forensic assessment, 150
    informed consent in, 105
    response validity in, 47–49, 156
Forensic referral sources, 92–94, 93*t*

Freud, Sigmund, 4–5
Fritsch, Gustav, 4
Functionalist approach, 10, 183
Future directions in clinical
        neuropsychology, 114–15
    advocacy, 118–21
    EBPP and outcomes focus, 121–23
    professional identity, 115–18, 116*f*, 117*f*

g. *See* General factor
Gait observation, 70
Galton, Francis, 5–6
GDS. *See* Geriatric Depression Scale
General factor (g), 6
Geriatric Depression Scale (GDS), 57
Gestalt approach, 34
    in clinical neuropsychology
        foundations, 11
    defined, 183
Goddard, Henry, 8
Goldstein, Kurt, 11
Group Examination Alpha, 8–9
Group Examination Beta, 8–9

Halstead, Ward, 10, 34–35
Halstead–Reitan Neuropsychological Test
        Battery (HRB)
    as assessment strategy, 35–37, 36*t*
    in clinical neuropsychology
        foundations, 10
    defined, 183
HC. *See* Houston Conference
Health care policy, 114–15
Heilbronner, Robert, 25
Hitzig, Eduard, 4
Houston Conference (HC), 95, 102
    clinical neuropsychologist defined, 135
    continuing education, 139
    defined, 183–84
    diversity in education and training, 140
    doctoral education, 138
    in education and training for clinical
        neuropsychology, 19–21
    internship training, 138
    introduction to, 134–35
    knowledge base, 135–36
    model of integrated education and
        training, 140–41, 140*f*
    persons needing clinical neuropsychology
        education and training, 135
    preamble for, 134
    professional and scientific activity, 135
    residency education and training,
        138–39
    skills, 136–38

subspecialities within clinical
  neuropsychology, 139
HRB. *See* Halstead–Reitan
  Neuropsychological Test Battery
Hypothesis testing approach. *See* Process
  approach

Idiographic knowledge, 44, 184
Independent Medical Evaluation (IME), 184
  consultation for, 91–94, 93t
Informed consent, 103–5, 149
INS. *See* International Neuropsychological
  Society
INS/Division 40 Task Force on Education,
  Accreditation, and
  Credentialing, 15–16, 102
  doctoral training program
    guidelines, 125–27
  internship guidelines, 127–28
  official report of, 125–30
  postdoctoral training guidelines, 128–30
Instruments. *See* Tests
Insurance providers, consultation
  with, 92–94, 93t
Integrated education and training, 140–41, 140f
Intellectual development, 6–7
Intellectual functioning assessment, 40t
Intelligence Quotient (IQ), 7, 184
Intelligence testing, 6–9
International Neuropsychological Society
  (INS), 14–16. *See also* INS/Division 40
  Task Force on Education, Accreditation,
  and Credentialing
Internships
  HC policy statement on, 138
  INS/Division 40 Task Force on Education,
    Accreditation, and Credentialing
    guidelines for, 127–28
Interorganizational Summit on Education
  and Training (ISET), 21
Interpretation, of tests, 157–59
Interpreters, 108–9, 152
Intervention and consultation, 85–86
  consultation with clinical referral
    sources, 90–92, 91t
  consultation with forensic referral
    sources, 92–94, 93t
  patient feedback and family
    consultation, 86–87
  psychotherapy with cognitively impaired
    individuals, 89–90
  rehabilitation psychology and cognitive
    rehabilitation, 87–89
  skills needed for, 137
  supervision roles, 95–96

teaching/educational roles, 94–95
Interview, of patient and significant
  others, 153–54
Iowa-Benton School of Neuropsychological
  Assessment, 39
IQ. *See* Intelligence Quotient
ISET. *See* Interorganizational Summit on
  Education and Training

Jackson, John Hughlings, 4

Knowledge
  idiographic, 44, 184
  nomothetic, 44–45, 184
  specialized, 132
Knowledge base, HC policy statement
  on, 135–36
Knox, Howard, 8–9

Language
  assessment of, 41t, 54
  observation of, 70–71
  test selection considerations and, 108–9,
    151–52
Learning/memory assessment, 41t, 54–55
Luria, Alexander, 11
Luria Nebraska Neuropsychological
  Battery, 37

Malingered neurocognitive dysfunction
  (MND), 50
Malingering, 47–50
Managed care practices, 114–15, 119
Measures. *See* Tests
Measurement. *See* Assessment
Memory. *See* Learning/memory
Mental age, 7
Methods. *See* Procedures
Minnesota Multiphasic Personality Inventory–
  2nd Edition (MMPI-2), 55, 57
MND. *See* Malingered neurocognitive
  dysfunction
Mood
  in neuropsychological evaluation
    report, 77–78
  observation of, 71
Mood disorders, 55–57
Motivation. *See* Effort
Motor functioning assessment, 41t
Movement observation, 70

National Academy of Neuropsychology (NAN)
  clinical neuropsychology defined
    by, 21–23, 142–43
  ethics policy statements of, 99–100

Neurology, history of, 4–5
Neuropsychological assessment. *See*
    Assessment
Neuropsychological evaluation report
    AACN practice guidelines statement
        on, 159–60
    behavioral observations in, 68–72
    collateral information in, 78
    content areas of, 66–67
    ethical considerations for, 109–10
    evaluation rationale in, 67–68
    patient background in, 67–68, 72–78
    recommendations in, 80–81
    record review in, 79
    referral source in, 67–68
    summary and diagnostic impressions
        in, 79–80
    test results in, 79
    writing for, 63–67
Nomothetic knowledge, 44–45, 184
Normative data, 53, 155

Observation. *See* Behavioral observations
Occupational history, in neuropsychological
    evaluation report, 74–75
Onset of complaint, in neuropsychological
    evaluation report, 73–74
Outcomes focus, 121–23
Outdated tests, 106

PAI. *See* Personality Assessment Inventory
Patient background
    ADLs, 74
    complaint onset and course, 73–74
    family history, 76
    mood and emotional functioning,
        77–78
    in neuropsychological evaluation
        report, 67–68, 72–78
    personal health, 76–77
    precipitating event, 72–73
    pre-morbid, 51–53
    psychiatric history, 76–77
    social, academic, and occupational
        history, 74–75
    subjective cognitive limitations, 73–74
Patient behaviors
    gait and movement, 70
    mood and affect, 71
    in neuropsychological evaluation
        report, 68–72
    presentation and demeanor, 69–70
    relationship to examiner, 71–72
    speech and language, 70–71
    task approach, 71–72

Patient feedback, 86–87
    AACN practice guidelines statement
        on, 160–61
    ethical considerations for, 112
Patient interview, 153–54
Pearson, Karl, 6
Pediatric neuropsychology, 30
Pediatric Neuropsychology Special Interest
    Group (PNSIG), 30
Performance tests, 8–9, 184
Personal health, in neuropsychological
    evaluation report, 76–77
Personality assessment, 56–57
Personality Assessment Inventory (PAI), 57
Physicians, consultation with, 90–92, 91*t*
Piaget, Jean, 7
PNSIG. *See* Pediatric Neuropsychology
    Special Interest Group
Population-based case
    conceptualization, 58–59
Populations served, in clinical
    neuropsychology, 27–29, 132
Postdoctoral training
    APPCN curriculum for, 96
    INS/Division 40 Task Force on Education,
        Accreditation, and Credentialing
        guidelines for, 128–30
Post-evaluation, ethical considerations
    during, 110–12
Practice guidelines, 23–26. *See also* AACN
    Practice Guidelines for
    Neuropsychological Assessment and
    Consultation; Ethical standards of practice
Precipitating event, in neuropsychological
    evaluation report, 72–73
Pre-evaluation, ethical considerations
    during, 100–103
Pre-morbid background, 51–53
Prescriptive authority, 93
Presentation, in neuropsychological
    evaluation report, 69–70
Probability distributions, 6, 184
Procedures, 133
    AACN practice guidelines statement
        on, 152–61
Process approach, 12, 34–35
Professional activity, HC policy statement
    on, 135
Professional alliances, 120–21
Professional identity, 115–18, 116*f*, 117*f*
Professional practice of clinical
    neuropsychology, 13
    consumer's perspective on, 23–26
    Division 40 work in, 15–19
    HC work in, 19–21

historical milestones in, 14*t*
INS work in, 14–16
NAN work in, 21–23
populations served in, 27–29, 132
problems addressed in, 26–27, 26*t*
subspecialization, 29–30, 139
Psychiatric history, in neuropsychological
    evaluation report, 76–77
Psychological functioning assessment, 55–57
Psychologists, consultation with, 90–92, 91*t*
Psychology, in clinical neuropsychology
    foundations, 6–7
Psychometrics, 5–12, 184
Psychotherapy, with cognitively impaired
    individuals, 89–90
Public description of clinical
    neuropsychology, 132–33

Qualitative approaches, 34, 45
Quantitative approaches, 34, 45

Race considerations, 107–9, 151–52
Recommendations, in neuropsychological
    evaluation report, 80–81
Record review, 153
    in neuropsychological evaluation
    report, 79
Referral question
    clarification of, 152
    ethical considerations for, 100–102
Referral source
    clarification of, 152
    consultation with, 90–94, 91*t*, 93*t*
    in neuropsychological evaluation
    report, 67–68
Rehabilitation psychology, 87–89
Reimbursement practices, 114–15, 119
Reitan, Ralph, 10, 35
Release of information, 110–12, 151
Reliability, of tests, 46–51, 107
Report writing, 63–65
    AACN practice guidelines statement
    on, 159–60
    effective strategies for, 65–67
    ethical considerations for, 109–10
Research skills, 137
Residency, HC policy statement on, 138–39
Response validity assessment, 42*t*, 46–51,
    55, 156
Revised tests, 106–7
Rey, Andre, 49

Scientific activity, HC policy statement on, 135
Scientific foundations of clinical
    neuropsychology, 3

clinical medicine influences, 4–5
intelligence testing, 6–9
neuropsychological assessment, 9–12
psychometric influences, 5–12
Scoring, of measurements, 157
Second opinions, 150–51
Security, of tests, 111–12, 151
Sensory functioning assessment, 41*t*, 55
Significant other. *See* Familiar other
Simon, Theodore, 6–7
Skills
    in clinical neuropsychology, 133, 136–38
    HC policy statement on, 136–38
Social history, in neuropsychological
    evaluation report, 74–75
Spearman, Charles, 6
Specialized knowledge, in clinical
    neuropsychology, 132
Speech
    assessment of, 41*t*, 54
    observation of, 70–71
Standardized batteries, 35–37, 36*t*
Standard measures, 51–52
Stanford–Binet scale, 7, 9
Stern, William, 7
Student supervision, neuropsychologist
    role in, 95–96
Subjective cognitive limitations, 73–74
Subspecialization
    in clinical neuropsychology, 29–30
    HC policy statement on, 139
Summary, in neuropsychological evaluation
    report, 79–80
Supervision
    neuropsychologist role in, 95–96
    skills needed for, 137–38
Symptom Validity Indices (SVIs), 42*t*, 49–50
Symptom Validity Testing (SVT), 42*t*,
    48–50, 184

Task approach, observation of, 71–72
Teaching. *See* Education and training
Technician supervision, neuropsychologist
    role in, 95–96
Terman, Lewis, 7
Tests, 43
    administration and scoring of, 157
    flexible battery approach, 35–37, 39–40,
    40*t*–42*t*
    interpretation of, 157–59
    reliability of, 46–51, 107
    security of, 111–12, 151
    selection of, 51–53, 105–9, 151–52
    standard, 51–52
    standardized batteries, 35–37, 36*t*

Test data, 111–12
Test materials, 111–12, 151
Test results, in neuropsychological evaluation
    report, 79
Teuber, Lukas, 11
Third-party assessments, 149–51
Training. *See* Education and training
Traumatic brain injury. *See* Brain injury
Treatment. *See* Intervention and consultation

Validity, 107, 152, 155–57, 159. *See also*
    Response validity assessment
Verbal fluency, 54
Visual-spatial function assessment, 41*t*

WAIS. *See* Wechsler Adult Intelligence Scale
Wechsler, David, 9

Wechsler Adult Intelligence Scale
    (WAIS), 37, 54–55
Wechsler Bellevue scale, 9
Wechsler Memory Scale (WMS), 106
Wechsler scales, 9–10
Wernicke, Karl, 4
Willis, Thomas, 4
WMS. *See* Wechsler Memory Scale
Work settings, AACN Practice Guidelines
    statement on, 148–49
Writing. *See* Report writing
Wundt, Wilhelm, 6, 10

Yerkes, Robert, 8–9

Zangwill, Oliver, 11

ABOUT THE AUTHORS

Greg J. Lamberty, PhD, ABPP is a clinical neuropsychologist with the Minneapolis VA Health Care System. He is the Rehabilitation/EC&R Psychology Supervisor, the site Project Director for Traumatic Brain Injury Model Systems and the Director of the Neuropsychology Postdoctoral Fellowship. Dr. Lamberty teaches graduate courses at the University of St. Thomas in Minneapolis and is an assistant professor in the Department of Psychiatry at the University of Minnesota Medical School. He has also held adjunct faculty positions at the University of Iowa, Purdue University, and the University of St. Thomas. Dr. Lamberty conducts clinical research in the assessment and treatment of patients with traumatic brain injury. He served on the Board of Directors of the American Academy of Clinical Neuropsychology (AACN) from 2002–2010 and was President from 2008–2010. Dr. Lamberty co-edited *The Practice of Clinical Neuropsychology* (2003) and wrote *Understanding Somatization in the Practice of Clinical Neuropsychology* (2008), also published by Oxford University Press.

Nathaniel W. Nelson, Ph.D., ABPP is is co-founder of Twin Cities Neuropsychology Partners, LLC and Assistant Professor of Psychology at University of St. Thomas, Graduate School of Professional Psychology. Dr. Nelson is actively involved in neuropsychology research and has published widely in peer-reviewed journals. His current research interests include symptom validity assessment, cognitive outcomes following mild traumatic brain injury, and psychological outcomes of traumatic brain injury as assessed by the Minnesota Multiphasic Personality Inventory-2-Restructured Form (RF). In addition to ongoing research activities at University of St. Thomas, Dr. Nelson collaborates as a research consultant with colleagues of the Minneapolis Veterans Health Care System and the University of Minnesota. He is a Member of the Editorial Board for *The Clinical Neuropsychologist*, a Consulting Editor for *Assessment*, and is co-head section editor of the Symptom Validity/Malingering section for *Psychological Injury and Law.* He is a licensed psychologist in the State of Minnesota, and is board-certified in clinical neuropsychology by the American Board of Professional Psychology.

ABOUT THE SERIES EDITORS

Arthur M. Nezu, Ph.D., ABPP is Professor of Psychology, Medicine, and Public Health at Drexel University and Special Professor of Forensic Mental Health and Psychiatry at the University at Nottingham in the United Kingdom. He is a fellow of multiple professional associations including the American Psychological Association, and board-certified by the American Board of professional Psychology in Cognitive and Behavioral Psychology, Clinical Psychology, and Clinical Health Psychology. Dr. Nezu is widely published, is incoming Editor of the *Journal of Consulting and Clinical Psychology*, and has maintained a practice for three decades.

Christine Maguth Nezu, Ph.D., ABPP, is Professor of Psychology and Medicine at Drexel University, and Special Professor of Forensic Mental Health and Psychiatry at the University at Nottingham in the United Kingdom. With over 25 years experience in clinical private practice, consultation/liaison, research, and teaching, Dr. Maguth Nezu is board-certified by the American Board of Professional Psychology (ABPP) in Cognitive and Behavioral Psychology and Clinical Psychology. She is also a past President of ABPP. Her research has been supported by federal, private, and state-funded agencies and she has served as a grant reviewer for the National Institutes of Health.

CPSIA information can be obtained at www.ICGtesting.com
Printed in the USA
BVOW012234190112

280819BV00004B/6/P